THE ESTHETICIAN'S GUIDE TO BUSINESS MANAGEMENT

HENRY J. GAMBINO, PH.D.

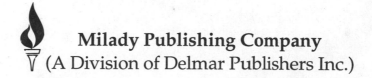
Milady Publishing Company
(A Division of Delmar Publishers Inc.)

NOTICE TO THE READER

Credits:

Administrative Editor:	Catherine Frangie
Developmental Editor:	Joseph Miranda
Senior Project Editor:	Laura Miller
Freelance Project Editor:	Pamela Fuller
Production Manager:	John Mickelbank
Art/Design Supervisor:	Susan Mathews

Copyright © 1994
Milady Publishing Company
(A Division of Delmar Publishers Inc.)

For information address:
3 Columbia Circle, Box 12519
Albany, NY 12212-2519

Printed in the United States of America.
Published simultaneously in Canada by Nelson Canada,
a division of the Thompson Corporation.

1 2 3 4 5 6 7 8 9 10 XXX 00 99 98 97 96 95 94

Library of Congress Cataloging-in-Publication Data

Gambino, Henry J.
   The esthetician's guide to business management / Henry J. Gambino.
      p.   cm.
   Includes index.
   ISBN 1-56253-127-1
   1. Beauty shops—Management. I. Title
TT965.G36 1994
646.7'2'068—dc20
                                                          93—4228
                                                            CIP

C O N T E N T S

iii

FOREWORD

With apologies to Charles Dickens, for the small business person, now is the best of times and the worst of times. Whether you are just starting in business or have been in operation for some time, you face many challenges. It is not easy to run a business successfully. You'll find there are many factors that affect your operation—external influences, such as the state of the economy and your competition, as well as internal influences, such as your ability to raise the capital you need and to provide quality services.

But you have many opportunities as well. To the extent you are able to overcome the external and internal influences, you control your own future. To a very great extent, how well you succeed is entirely up to you. But you have to be up to the task of running your esthetics salon business. That means you have to be more than just a competent practitioner of the profession. You have to think and act like a business person. And that takes planning, expertise, and knowledge of a great many subjects beyond esthetics.

This book helps you acquire the knowledge you need to run your salon successfully. Chapter 1 provides an overview of business. Note the discussion on why businesses fail or succeed. The mortality rate for new businesses is very high. If you understand the reasons businesses fail, you'll be better able to avoid the pitfalls. This chapter also makes you look inward, at yourself and your motivations for being in business for yourself.

Chapter 2 discusses the business plan, the most important document you will prepare for your salon. Without a well-thought-out, comprehensive plan for your business, your chances of success are slim indeed. Chapter 3 describes the different forms of organization your salon business can take and outlines the advantages and disadvantages of each. It also covers what you need to know if you purchase an existing salon or buy a franchise operation. Chapters 4 and 5 help you decide which services to offer in your esthetics salon and how to develop an effective salon design.

Then there's the law. Any business faces a number of regulatory and tax liability pressures and your esthetics salon is no different. Chapters 6 and 7 describe the various federal, state, and local government agencies that will affect your business and discuss their various requirements.

As you run your esthetics salon, you will quickly learn the importance of money in business. You need it; you can't operate without it. Chapter 8 discusses your capital requirements and how to acquire the money you need. Chapter 9 shows you how to keep track of the money that comes in and goes out. It also covers budgeting, pricing, and control of expenses.

The balance of the book deals with the day-to-day operations of your salon. Chapter 10 discusses how to find, hire, and keep qualified help. Chapter 11 discusses how to determine your equipment and supply requirements, how to purchase those items, and how to institute inventory controls. Chapters 12 and 13 cover salon operations, handling various client types, and retail sales. Chapter 14 tells you how to computerize your salon. In this technological age, a computer system is a virtual necessity.

No matter how good your services are, you won't have any business unless prospective clients know you exist. Chapter 15 expresses the importance of advertising and promotion. This chapter discusses planning and execution of advertising programs and covers the various media you should or shouldn't consider.

Sanitation and safety in your salon are always of concern. That is the province of Chapter 16. By this time, however, you are probably almost in despair as you realize how much you have to know and how varied that knowledge must be. Well, you needn't lose heart. There is a lot of help available for small business people, and Chapter 17 tells you where to get it.

There is nothing revolutionary or startling in this book. The work contains sound business practices and techniques that have been proved effective. Just remember, however, that there are no guarantees in business. You may follow all of these principles to the letter and still fail. By the same token, you may disregard them and still succeed. There is always an element of luck involved. But your chances of success are markedly better if you know and practice these principles of good business.

Arm yourself with knowledge, summon up your courage, and go out and face the world of business. Congratulations. You are now an entrepreneur. And good luck.

HJG, Doylestown, Pennsylvania, 1993

ACKNOWLEDGMENTS

A book may list only one author, but there are many people involved in its making. This book is certainly no exception. I would like to thank all those people who helped turn this book from an idea into a reality. First, very special thanks to Joseph M. Sherlock, one of the most astute small businessmen I know, who patiently reviewed every chapter and whose advice and suggestions helped make this book better. Thanks also go to other experts who have reviewed specific chapters whose suggestions were equally valuable. These people are Louis Peirera, a financial analyst, and Thomas Cronin, an accountant, who reviewed the financial information; Clifford W. Keevan and John R. Gill, both experienced advertising experts, who reviewed the chapter on advertising and promotion; and J. McCullagh, a computer expert, who checked the accuracy of the chapter on computers.

Finally, I'd like to extend a very special thanks to my wife, Maureen, who patiently proofread every page of the book and made numerous suggestions on style and grammar, and without whose support and encouragement I could not have completed the project.

INTRODUCTION TO THE
ESTHETICS BUSINESS

C H A P T E R

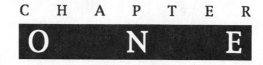

Congratulations! You have decided to open your own skin care salon, or you've recognized the need to manage your existing salon more efficiently. You are entering into the world of small business. You have become an entrepreneur. According to *Webster's Ninth New Collegiate Dictionary*, an entrepreneur is "one who organizes, manages and assumes the risks of a business or enterprise." Many people feel that an entrepreneur is a risk-taker. There is a considerable element of risk in starting any new business or even in managing an established business, but a successful entrepreneur is not a risk-taker. Rather, he or she is a risk-recognizer and a risk-manager. That is, he or she is aware of the risks and, through proper and prudent management, minimizes their potential effect.

You are starting a journey on which you will go where many have gone before—and where most have failed. Make no mistake. Starting and managing a successful business is difficult. It takes skill, knowledge, perseverance, hard work, and a considerable amount of luck. And there are no guarantees of success. The failure rate for new businesses is high. More than half of all new businesses don't make it past the first five years. Many of those go under in the first year.

WHY BUSINESSES FAIL

There are many reasons a business can fail. The majority just don't make enough money. They can't pay their bills. They don't earn a living for the owner. Then they fold. Face this fact right up front. The purpose of a business is to make a profit. You have to earn money. There's nothing wrong with that. Our economy depends on businesses making profits, earning income, providing others with jobs. Those profits return to the economy. If you don't make enough profit to pay all your business expenses and to let you live in the lifestyle you choose, you won't be successful.

A sizeable portion fail because they start with insufficient capital. They don't have enough cash at the outset to see them through the hard times at the beginning. They can't afford to acquire the equipment, the facilities or the supplies they need to carry their business to success, or build up so much debt, they can't meet their obligations. And they go under.

Inexperience in managing a business is another reason companies fail. The owners just don't know what they're doing. Take yourself, for example. You are undoubtedly a competent esthetician or cosmetologist, fully capable of performing the services you are considering offering. (If you're not, you should be practicing those skills, not thinking about starting your own skin care salon.) But no matter how good you are at your profession, you are not automatically qualified to run a business. You have to think like a business person, not like an esthetician. You have to be aware of good management practices, and you have to put them to use.

Inability to manage expenses is also a cause of many business failures. Many small business owners don't control their expenses and their cash flow so they quickly run into financial trouble and can't recover. Or they let their overhead expenses run uncontrolled until they're buried by their operating costs. Their costs go so high they can't make a profit, even though they enjoy a good volume of business. You must manage your costs. Good financial management is vital to business success.

Some businesses fail because the industry in which they operate gets weak. This is why many businesses fail during a recession or a downturn in the economy. As the economy goes down, people stop buying the products and services, and the businesses lose money. You might think there's nothing you can do about this. It's just the breaks. But you would be wrong. Businesses that are well managed have the ability to weather industry weakness and survive, even prosper, when their competition fails.

CHECKLIST 1-1
REASONS BUSINESSES FAIL

Businesses fail for many reasons:

1. Failure to generate sufficient income
2. Insufficient capital
3. Inexperience in business management
4. Inability to manage expenses
5. Recessions or weaknesses in the industry

WHY BUSINESSES SUCCEED

Businesses succeed because they are managed properly. The owners know what they are doing. They control as many of the variables as possible and reduce as many risks as they can. They recognize their own strong and weak points and work within their limitations. They dare to dream, but they don't fantasize. They live within the realities of the business and economic world they inhabit.

The owners of successful businesses start with sufficient capital. They can acquire the things they need to perform the necessary business functions, advertise and promote the business properly, and meet their expenses. And they have enough cash reserves to last until the business starts earning profits.

The owners succeed because they control their costs and expenses. They purchase only what they need, don't waste their resources, follow sound financial practices, and keep accurate, complete records. They analyze their businesses constantly. They know which products and services are profitable and which aren't and change their product or service mix to fit the profit picture.

Businesses are successful because their owners work hard. They put in the hours necessary to accomplish everything that has to be done. Successful business owners do their homework. They learn what they must and get the proper training. They have a good sense

**CHECKLIST 1-2
REASONS BUSINESSES SUCCEED**

Businesses succeed because the owners:

1. Manage them properly.
2. Control all possible variables.
3. Manage risks well.
4. Have sufficient capital.
5. Control costs and expenses adequately.
6. Don't waste resources.
7. Put in the hard work and long hours necessary.
8. Are tough and resilient.
9. Can make hard decisions based on facts.
10. Use common sense.
11. Have good people skills.
12. Recognize the importance of their customers.
13. Have a vision and goals.

of what they can do themselves and what they must hire others to do, and hire experts where experts are needed.

The owners or managers are tough, resilient people who persevere even when times are tough. They don't quit. They have the ability to look at the facts and make hard decisions, even when those decisions may be unpopular or contrary to their desires. They exercise good common sense.

Successful business owners have good people skills and know how to handle employees. They hire the right people, train them properly, motivate them, and treat them fairly. In return, they earn the loyalty of their staff members, who will often give that little extra that can mean the difference between success and failure.

Most of all, successful business owners recognize the importance of their customers. These owners know they will be successful only if their customers are satisfied. They give quality, service, and value for the dollars the customers give them. They build a loyal customer base. Their clients return again and again and recommend the business to their friends and neighbors. But the owners don't rest on that customer base. They try constantly to expand it and bring new clients into the business by marketing, advertising, and promoting their products and services to keep their name before existing and future customers. They understand the first principle of marketing: businesses exist to meet customer needs. They know their customers buy product or service benefits, not product or service features. They know what their customers want and do everything they can to satisfy those wants.

Successful entrepreneurs have a vision that they translate into goals. They develop a comprehensive plan of action to reach those goals and are not afraid to implement that plan.

THE ESTHETICS BUSINESS

Esthetics, the nonmedical care of the skin, is a growing part of the health and beauty industry. Skin, that marvelous living fabric that covers and protects the human body, requires ongoing care to keep it healthy and beautiful. The integument is subjected daily to a wide range of stress and harm. Environmental pollution, airborne dirt, and exposure to the ultraviolet radiation of sunlight all combine to damage skin, as do many other factors, such as the effects of smoking, exposure to chemicals, failure to properly cleanse the skin, poor diet, and aging. And in our fast-paced society, people don't have, or don't take, the time to properly cleanse and care for their skin.

More and more, people recognize the importance of good skin care, but they lack the knowledge to take care of their skin themselves. They are bombarded with advertising and promotions for a variety of products sold over-the-counter in department or specialty stores or by mail order. Some of these products are good; they work and are effective. But many promise much more than they can deliver. People may be able to buy products for their skin but are not getting the advice and care they need. They require professional help—from an esthetician working in a licensed skin care salon.

There is a market for skin care and related services. Just look at the media's interest in the subject and the wealth of products in the stores. Virtually every woman's magazine regularly features articles on skin and body care, along with the myriad of advertisements for skin care products. The manufacturers of these products are spending millions of dollars on advertising and promotion to capitalize on this interest. And it's working. The sales of retail skin care products run into the billions of dollars each year.

Nor is the market limited to women. In ever-increasing numbers, men are becoming aware of the need to care for their skin. Men's skin is just as subject to damage from the effects of pollution, smoking, and associated hazards. Skin care is for everyone, regardless of sex, ethnic background, or age.

The market potential is huge. There is a niche for well-equipped skin and body care salons staffed with well-trained estheticians and support people where clients can get effective, competent care for their skin, along with advice on maintaining their skin in good health. But success is not automatic. Salons that succeed will be those that correctly identify their target audiences, market their services properly to that audience, locate in a place accessible to those customers, develop a loyal base of repeat customers, and manage the business effectively, using sound management practices.

The beauty business, of which skin care salons are a part, is a more personal enterprise than other kinds of business, such as sales or manufacturing. Much depends on the interplay and amity between buyer and seller. But even so, the salon business is still governed by the same management principles as other businesses.

That the successful esthetics salons must provide top-quality services is a given. No matter how well managed the salon may be from the business aspects, without the ability to deliver quality services, there's no chance of success. But quality services alone don't guarantee success. They only let the salons compete in the marketplace.

REASONS FOR GETTING INTO BUSINESS

So, you want to open your own skin care salon. Why? That's an important question. There are a lot of reasons for going into business for yourself. All may be good, but some are better than others. Whatever your reasons, make sure you understand just what you're getting into.

Do you want to be your own boss? Do you want to be independent? They're admirable reasons. No one will tell you what to do. You have to answer to no one. But you will find that, in effect, a lot of people will be telling you what to do. Your customers will be demanding quality, value, and satisfaction. Your banker will be demanding payment of loans along with periodic reporting. The government wants taxes and records of your transactions on time and according to schedule. Your employees expect work and pay. Your creditors want to be paid for supplies, equipment, and services. You'll sometimes feel as though you answer to everyone. Being the boss entails a lot of responsibility. You are responsible for everything that happens in your salon, from the safety and earning power of your employees to paying the bills. But you are the one in charge. Everyone will look to you to make the right decisions.

Do you want to escape from the daily nine-to-five routine? Are you looking to get away from the humdrum and boredom of a job? When you own your own salon, you will not be bored. You won't have time. Often, you'll feel overwhelmed by the amount and complexity of all the things you have to do (running the day-to-day operations, finding capital, long-range planning) and all of the people with whom you'll have to deal (bankers, employees, customers, accountants, lawyers, sales people). You'll be amazed at the amount of detail you will have to consider; things you were never concerned with when you worked for someone else. Nor will you have to worry about the eight-hour workday. Now, you will put in twelve to eighteen or more hours every day, seven days a week. Even when your salon is closed, you'll be busy. But, in spite of the work and the hours, you'll have the satisfaction of knowing that you're doing it for yourself. The rewards are yours.

Do you want to make more money and better your standard of living? Owning your own business can do that, but it's not guaranteed. You may be only marginally successful and earn just enough profit to get by. And, there is the very real possibility you will lose everything. The hard work you put in may not translate to more dollars for you, but it can happen if you manage the business correctly. It is up to you to make the right decisions and do the right things.

Do you want the prestige of being a business owner? Do you want the satisfaction of being on your own? There is prestige in being a successful entrepreneur. You will attain some degree of status in your community, but you'll have to work hard for it. And there is great satisfaction in building something that works well. That satisfaction is made even sweeter when you have to work to earn it.

Do you believe you can provide skin and body care services better than anyone else and want to offer those services to the community? That is a necessary attitude. If you don't think you are better than the competition, you will be hard pressed to succeed. If you can't offer something better to your prospective customers, there's no reason for them to patronize your salon. Granted, you're in business to earn a profit, but it is an honest profit, based on providing quality services and value to your clientele. You must be willing to give your very best. If you are getting into business just for the fast buck, you haven't a chance.

QUALIFICATIONS FOR GETTING INTO BUSINESS

Opening your own salon requires a number of personal, professional, and technical qualifications. You have to take stock of yourself and assure you have what it takes to be a successful business person.

Personal Qualifications

The personal qualities you bring to the task are most important and are necessary to your success. You have to examine yourself carefully and honestly. Are you a people person? When you are in business for yourself, you will deal with many different people—customers, employees, tradespeople, and many more. You must have the ability to negotiate with these people and to get along with them. And that's hard to do unless you genuinely like people.

Are you a decision maker? Do you have the ability to analyze facts and make sound judgments? Management means making intelligent choices from a sometimes limited list of options and resources; it means setting priorities and making compromises. You must be able to do that. You must also have the ability to plan ahead, to look forward and make decisions that move your business in the direction you want it to go. You have to be pro-active, not re-active. You can't wait for situations to develop, then react to them. You must anticipate them, and act before problems arise.

Do you have the mental and emotional toughness you need? There is a tremendous strain involved in operating a business. You have to be tough enough to stand up to the mental roller coaster of business—the highs and the lows. Can you keep things in perspective? You have to be able to look at things objectively, to be capable of

CHECKLIST 1-3
BUSINESS QUALIFICATIONS

Personal Qualifications:

1. Be a people person.
2. Be a decision-maker.
3. Be mentally and emotionally tough.
4. Enjoy challenges.
5. Have the support of your family and/or significant other.
6. Be physically capable.

Professional Qualifications:

1. Be a competent practitioner of all services offered.
2. Understand the theory and practice of all services.
3. Be willing to stay current on trends in the field.
4. Participate in trade associations.

Technical Qualifications:

1. Understand business aspects.
2. Be able to manage finances.
3. Be a capable organizer and planner.
4. Be a capable personnel manager.
5. Know how to deal effectively with customers.
6. Be aware of all applicable laws and regulations.
7. Understand advertising and promotion.
8. Know where to get the help you need.

stepping back and assessing the situation dispassionately, without letting your emotions cloud your judgment. You have to stay calm, cool, and collected in the face of crises, both big and small. And it helps if you have a sense of humor. Take your business very seriously, but don't take yourself too seriously. Try to have fun; it makes everything easier.

Do you have the physical stamina and strength to operate the business? You have to be in good health to withstand the strain, the hard work, and the long hours you'll put into the business. You have to ride through the aches, the pains, and the fatigue you will often feel. Your body has to be able to stand up to long days and short nights, often for prolonged periods of time.

Do you like challenges? Owning your own business is a challenge. You have to like facing the day-to-day demands of business. You have to attack them head-on, not shy away from them. If you don't face them squarely, they will overwhelm you. Do you enjoy competition? The esthetics salon business is highly competitive. There are many salons in business, each offering the same services, and presumably the same quality, as you. Competition can be a strain, but it can also be a challenge, especially if you enjoy the battle.

Do you have the support you need from your family or significant other? This is most important. With the long hours and the emotional and physical strains you face, you won't have much time for them, at least over the short run. And the financial burdens you face may mean a temporarily lower standard of living for them as well as for yourself. If they understand and support you, it will make those strains much easier to bear.

Professional Qualifications

To succeed in your skin and beauty care business, you must be a competent and able performer. You have to know the theory and practice of each and every service you offer in the salon. You have to know what steps are taken in each service and why. You have to know what equipment and supplies are needed and what facilities are required.

Do you have the professional skills you need? Do you have a thorough understanding of each and every service? Can you answer all your customers' questions? Can you separate the benefits of the services from the features? Can you train your employees? If you don't have these skills, consider acquiring them before you think about opening your own business. They are vital to your ability to offer quality services to your customers. You can't rely on the skills of your employees to carry your business. Certainly it's important to hire skilled help, but employees leave. You are the only truly permanent factor in your salon. It is up to you to be the expert.

As busy as you will be in managing your salon, you must also take the time to stay current in your field. That means you must be aware of new developments in esthetics, new products, and new techniques. You must have the interest to keep reading the trade magazines and new books on the subject, and to keep attending the trade shows. You should also join and be active in the local chapters of your trade associations.

Technical Qualifications

Being technically qualified means that you know about the business aspects of your company, the management principles, the finance and accounting functions, the employment functions, et al. When you own and operate your own business, you wear many hats. You will be much more than just a practitioner of your profession. You will also be a business manager. You'll be concerned with profit margins and income, with attracting new business, with the legal aspects of running a business, with the liabilities involved, and many other things.

There are many things you have to know, many skills you have to master, both to start your business and to operate it once you've opened your doors. You must be an organizer and a planner. You need to start with a sound, reasonable, well-thought-out business plan. Then you have to decide on your business organization.

Once you have decided which services you will offer, you must become a salon designer so you can work in the most efficient facility available to you. You have to be a personnel manager so you can hire the best people to work for you. And you have to learn how to become an effective employer to get the most from your staff. You have to manage your equipment and supplies to get the best, most cost-effective materials you need to operate successfully.

You have to know how to handle your customers. You will deal with all types of customers, each of which takes different handling. You will have to develop salon policies and procedures and set the standards under which your salon will operate. And you will have to enforce those standards.

Don't forget the law. You have to become aware of all the laws and regulations that govern salons and that apply to business in general. You also have to be aware of the risks and liabilities you may incur and be conversant with insurance requirements. Then there are the tax laws. You have to be aware of the taxes for which you are responsible on the federal, state, and local levels. And you have to be concerned with the health and safety aspects of your salon.

Another important set of responsibilities covers the financial aspects. You must know how to manage your cash, how to acquire the capital you need, and how to deal with bankers. You need to keep accurate and honest records, both to satisfy government requirements and for your own analysis and use.

You have to understand advertising and promotion, so you can market your services properly. No matter how good your services may be, you won't get customers to come into the salon unless you let them know you're there.

There is much you need to know when you operate your own business. Fortunately, a lot of help is available to you. You will hire competent people to handle some of these things, for example, an accountant to help you with the financial aspects of the business and with your taxes, an attorney to help you with the legal aspects, an insurance agent to help you protect your business, etc. But you have to know enough about all of these things to discuss them intelligently with the people you hire. You have to be willing to learn those things you don't know, even though you may have to expend considerable time and effort to acquire that knowledge.

THE BUSINESS OF BUSINESS

Business success or failure doesn't depend on whether you are male or female, on your ethnic background, on your education. It depends on your ability, intelligence, and willingness to work. You, and no one else, will have to manage your business. You have to utilize good management practices.

You also need a certain amount of good luck, although in business, luck is largely a matter of preparation. Keep in mind that there are no guarantees. Even if you do everything right, you can still fail. You want to control as many variables as possible, but you can't control them all. There will always be some element of risk involved. Your goal is to minimize that risk.

Remember, no one is as interested in your business as you are. If you won't make the sacrifices necessary to learn what you need to know, to do what you must do, no one will do it for you. You have to put in the work, make the decisions, and take the risks. But, in return, you get the rewards and the satisfaction of having created a successful business. It's all up to you.

SUMMARY

Starting your own business can be a risky venture. To be successful, you must learn to manage those risks. It takes hard work, perseverance, knowledge, and a measure of luck.

Most new businesses don't last five years. They fail for a number of reasons. They don't make enough profit to pay their bills and provide a reasonable lifestyle for the owner. Many fail because they don't have enough capital to purchase equipment and supplies or to properly promote the businesses. They don't have enough cash to last through the hard, lean times at the beginning. By the same token, many fail because the owners have no experience in running a business and make too many mistakes or do not control their expenses properly. Others fail because of downturns in the economy, which affect their ability to generate income.

Successful businesses, however, succeed because they are properly managed and sufficiently capitalized. Their owners manage risks effectively and live within the realities of their business world. And their owners put in the hard work and the long hours necessary. They know how to attract and keep customers and how to hire and motivate their employees. They understand that their businesses exist to meet customers' needs.

There are many reasons for getting into business: to be your own boss, to be independent, to escape the nine-to-five life, to increase your standard of living. These are all good reasons, but they all come with responsibilities. The fact is, you will work harder, longer hours and assume greater risk, with no more guarantee of success than if you work for someone else. But your potential rewards and satisfaction will be greater.

Getting into your own business requires a number of qualifications. The personal qualities include being a people person, with the ability to get along with all kinds of personalities and to make sound decisions based on facts and not on emotions. You also must be both mentally and physically tough to withstand the strain the venture can place on you. Professionally, you must be a competent and knowledgeable performer in your skin and body care services. Technically, from the business standpoint, you must understand and apply sound business principles.

Owning and operating your own skin and body care business is difficult and demanding. But if you have what it takes, personally, professionally, and technically, and are willing to persevere and do what is necessary, the rewards can be outstanding.

THE BUSINESS PLAN

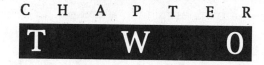

C H A P T E R

T W O

There is an old adage in business that says, to fail to plan is to plan to fail. In your venture, whether it's new or has existed for some time, no single element will be more important than your business plan. It is the first thing you should consider and develop once you've made the decision to open your own salon or to begin managing your existing salon in a more businesslike manner. Preparing a proper, complete, and well-written business plan makes you ask, and answer, the hard questions. It makes you take stock of yourself and your abilities, and it makes you aware of your shortcomings. It makes you do your homework.

You will also need your business plan when you apply for financing or credit. Few banks or commercial lending institutions will consider your application if you do not have a complete business plan that lets them know you have carefully thought out all aspects of your venture.

WHAT IS A BUSINESS PLAN?

Just as an architect develops a blueprint to build a house, you develop a business plan as the blueprint from which you will build your business. It is your detailed design, which sets out the goals you want to accomplish and how you expect to accomplish them. The business plan is the written expression of your hopes and dreams, but it is tempered with reality.

The business plan is a living, dynamic document. It takes a lot of time, thought, and effort to develop, and once you've developed the plan, you'll be constantly revising it. As your goals change, you will alter your business plan to keep up with those changes.

THE ELEMENTS OF THE BUSINESS PLAN

The business plan can be divided into two major segments, the nonfinancial aspects of the business and the financial aspects. The nonfinancial portion deals with your goals and ambitions, both short term and long term. It also examines items such as the competitive situation, the demographics of your customer base, the services you might offer, your strengths, and your weaknesses. This part of the plan puts your vision into words.

The financial part of the plan discusses how much your dreams will cost and where you are going to get the money to pay for them. While the nonfinancial part of the plan lets you exercise your vision, this part forces you to be realistic. And here, you must be realistic. It is very easy to underestimate your financial needs at this point. It is also very tempting to overestimate them, to add a "fudge factor" to cover incomplete planning. You do yourself no favor by under or overestimating your financial requirements. Either extreme will distort your needs and make them harder to fulfill.

Nonfinancial Elements

Your business plan starts with a mission statement. This is a declaration that describes what type of business you envision. It should be brief, but should also clearly state the purpose of your salon. What type of salon do you anticipate operating? It's not enough to say, for example, "The mission of this salon is to provide skin care services." Rather, a more accurate mission statement would say something like, "The mission of this salon is to provide a full range of professional skin and body care services, including facials, massage, waxing, electrology, and manicuring services to women within a fifteen-mile radius of the salon."

CHECKLIST 2-1
THE BUSINESS PLAN

Nonfinancial Elements:

1. Mission statement–a brief, clear statement of the purpose of your salon.
2. Brief biography of yourself and partners–an honest evaluation of your background.
   A. Education.
   B. Training
   C. Experience in business.
3. The competitive situation–data about the salons in the area with which you will compete.
   A. Locations.
   B. Traffic flow.
   C. Services they offer.
   D. Pricing.
4. Demographic data–information about your prospective customers.
   A. Who they are.
   B. How many there are.
   C. What services they want.
   D. Profile of your model customer.
5. Statement of your goals–a brief, clear declaration of what you want to accomplish with your business.
   A. Be specific.
   B. Be attainable.
   C. Be measurable.

Financial Elements:

1. Physical facilities–an examination of the premises you will occupy.
   A. Location
   B. Size
   C. Rent or mortgage amount
   D. Suitability for use
   E. Costs of utilities and services
   F. Costs of renovations
   G. Signage

2. Capital and noncapital equipment–an examination of the machinery and other apparatus you will need to provide the services you offer as well as what you need for the administration of the business.
    A. Equipment requirements
    B. Sources of the equipment
    C. Costs of the equipment
3. Supplies–an examination of the various supplies you will need to provide the services and maintain the business.
    A. Supply requirements
    B. Sources of the supplies
    C. Costs of the supplies
4. Staffing requirements–an examination of the number and type of employees you will need.
    A. Number of employees needed
    B. Cost of salaries
    C. Cost of benefits
5. Services–an examination of the services you will have to purchase to conduct your business.
    A. List of services needed
    B. Source of the services
    C. Costs of the services
6. Advertising and promotion–an examination of the type and amount of advertising and promotion you will have to do at the start of business operations.
    A. Advertising and promotion messages
    B. Advertising and promotion media
    C. Costs of advertising and promotion
7. Preliminary budget–an examination of the money requirements based on estimated costs for all items.
    A. Fixed, recurring expenses
    B. One-time expenses
8. Time lines–an examination of time parameters for accomplishing each task.
9. Source of money–an examination of where the money you require will come from.
    A. Money on hand
        1. Savings
        2. Other assets

> B. Personal loans
>   1. From bank
>   2. From credit cards
>   3. From friends or relatives
> C. Business loans
>   1. From banks
>   2. From other financial institutions
> D. Collateral
> **10.** Financial statement–a list of assets and liabilities.

Short and to the point? Yes, but it clearly and concisely sets the parameters of your business and focuses your attention on the details that will help make your salon a success. Each of the elements in the mission statement will be expanded upon in the balance of the business plan. The statement may also change as you continue to develop the document. As you elaborate on the other elements, you may have new ideas that will alter the mission. Don't be afraid to make those changes when they are warranted.

Let's examine just what the mission statement for this hypothetical salon has accomplished. First, it has described the kind of salon the owner wishes to operate. He or she wants to give facials, manicures, and related services. Next, it has indicated the customer base. He or she wants to offer these services primarily to women. Finally, it delimits the area of the business. Those women will be found mostly within a fifteen-mile radius of the salon.

Next, write a brief biography of yourself and your partners, if you have any. What is your education and training? Your background and experience? What makes you qualified to run the business you've chosen? Why do you think you'll be successful? This section will accomplish two things. First, it will let you know whether you're ready to go into business for yourself. It will start to uncover your weak points and your strong points. Second, it will help your banker make a determination of your qualifications when you apply for financing. Be honest with yourself. State your qualifications factually and fairly. And keep an open mind. You may be surprised at what you'll find out about you.

Under education, list your formal schooling, such as high school, college, and occupational training. List special subjects you may have studied, professional seminars you've attended, and manufacturer's classes you have gone to. Think about which subjects interested you the most and in which you did best. Also, look at the subjects that interested you the least and in which you did poorly. Look at the direction your education has taken you. You may find, for example, that you are highly trained in one or more aspects of cosmetology but are weak in others. It may also point out that you have no training in business management or that you have more than you thought.

Look at your experience. How long have you worked in the field? What experience have you had that will enable you to operate a business successfully? What experience outside of cosmetology have you had? This may include working in a retail store as a salesperson or working in an office. Experience is one of the most important factors in operating a business. That means experience in both providing the services and managing the salon. Length of time practicing as an esthetician or cosmetologist is not necessarily important. What matters is how you've learned and grown throughout your career.

Examine your biography. Does it indicate you have the knowledge and experience you need to succeed in business? Or does it suggest areas in which you need further study? Based on your biography, can you fulfill the mission of your salon? If the answer is "no," think about where you can get the knowledge you need. There are many sources of information, ranging from books to adult evening classes in management techniques.

Your business plan should also consider the competitive situation in the area in which you intend to operate. Survey the area. Count how many skin care salons are there. Look at the services they offer, the prices they charge, and their clientele. Check if the salons seem busy and if the work they do is adequate. If possible, talk to some of the owners. Talk to some of the customers. Get as much information as you can.

There's nothing illegal or unethical about gathering competitive intelligence. It's a necessary step in the process of establishing a business, but it requires considerable effort. You'll have to physically go and look at the situation. The information you obtain will tell you a lot and will help you make informed decisions. You may find out, for example, that all of the salons in the area are performing one type of service you will offer, but only a few offer other types you're planning. That may give you a competitive edge in those services. But, be aware that it may also mean there's no call for those services.

Knowing the prices other salons charge will give you some idea of how much you'll be able to charge. The average prices of services will show you what the clientele in the neighborhood is accustomed to paying. That doesn't mean you can't charge more, but you will need a good reason to get the higher dollars. It also doesn't mean you can't charge less, but if you do, you may be throwing earnings away.

Having an idea of the general traffic flow of the other salons will give you an idea of the level of business they enjoy. Although it will tell you whether the salons are busy, it won't necessarily tell you how profitable they are. It is possible to be busy and not make any money, although busy salons do generally make a profit. What the information will really tell you is the overall level of business available in the area. It should also give you an idea of the types of customers available, their age groups, their tastes, what kinds of services they prefer. This information is important when you work on your demographic data.

The competitive intelligence you gather, once analyzed, should provide you with a wide range of insights on business possibilities in your area of interest. If you note that a few salons are doing well and others doing poorly, examine the successful ones. Look at their location, their services, their prices; try to identify the reasons for their success. Conversely, look at the less successful salons. Analyze what they're doing and try to identify the reasons for their failure. Learn as much as you can from other people's accomplishments and mistakes. Keep an open mind and look for opportunities you may not have thought of before. What you find out may prompt you to revise your original mission statement.

Demographic data, which describes the characteristics of the people living and working in the area with which you're concerned, also belongs in your business plan. It will tell you who your potential customers are, how many of them there are, and what they want or need in the way of your services. How many people are in the area? Where do they live? What are their ages? Are they male or female? Married or single? How many children do they have? What are their occupations? What are their tastes? This type of information is available from a number of sources. The U. S. Government Census Bureau provides population breakdowns by age, sex, and household. The data is available in your local library or from the Government Printing Office and bookstores. Local newspapers and real estate offices are also good sources of demographic data in specific localities. You can also learn much through observation, for example at local shopping malls and supermarkets.

You have identified the kinds of customers you want to service in your mission statement. Now, you have to characterize them. Just who is going to patronize your salon and give you money in exchange for the services you plan to offer? Create a profile of your model customer. The profile should incorporate all of the characteristics you would like to see in your clients. For example, let's say you feel your ideal customer should be female, twenty-four to thirty-eight years old, white-collar worker, who dresses well and is interested in her appearance. She may be either single or married. She earns enough money to afford the services you will offer at the prices you will charge. Now, based on the demographic data you've gathered, how many people either living or working in the area fit that profile? How many of them can you reasonably expect to patronize your salon? Are there enough potential customers to let you earn enough profit to keep your business in operation?

You may find that there are not enough customers in the area to support your operation. In that case, you will have to either expand the area in which you intend to operate or widen your customer profile to include more people. As with most parts of the business plan, this information may lead you to revise your original mission statement.

You must also consider why these people should patronize your business. What will you offer that the competition doesn't? How will you reach these people? What message will you use to convince them to try your services, especially if they are satisfied with the services they're getting elsewhere?

A statement of your goals is also in order in this part of your business plan. This is different from your mission statement, which is a declaration of purpose. Your goals are a declaration of measurable accomplishment, both in the short term and the long term. Simply put, where do you want to be one year from now? Five years from now? Ten years from now? It is vitally necessary to consider these goals. How can you plan on reaching your destination if you don't know where you're going? This is the place to state your dreams and aspirations, especially for the long-term goals. Your short-term goals should be somewhat more realistic than the long-term goals. Both, however, should be specific, attainable, and measurable. That is, you should have a definite end in mind, and it should be possible to reach that end. And there should be some way to measure when you've reached it.

A poor short-term goal might be stated as follows: "By next year, I want to service a lot of customers and make $500,000 a year." This statement is not very specific. What constitutes a lot of customers? How do you measure it? Nor is the goal attainable. It is highly unrealistic to expect such a high return after only one year of operation. An example of a good short-term goal, however, might be stated: "One year from opening the salon, I expect the salon to have gross revenues of $100,000 per year, based on an average gross of $38.50 per client visit, and to earn a net profit of $6,000 after paying all expenses, including my salary." A long-term goal might state: "Ten years from opening, I want to have a chain of three salons offering a full range of skin and body care services. I expect to employ a total of twenty-five people. I expect each salon to earn $125,000 a year in gross revenues." These goals are specific, attainable, and measurable.

Will the goals be reached? There's no guarantee of that. Success depends on a combination of hard work, perseverance, good management, and a measure of luck. Are they worthwhile? That's strictly a matter of judgment. Goals will differ among individuals. What is a valid goal for one person will not be to another. But, no matter what your goals are, they give you something to reach for.

Financial Elements

The financial elements of your business plan concern the more tangible physical aspects, including such items as location, equipment, supplies, staffing, and services you'll have to purchase. This part of the business plan makes you look at what you need to accomplish your mission and meet your goals, where you are going to acquire those items, and how you're going to pay for them. It will also include your preliminary budget and time lines, and will help you establish contingency plans. An examination of the financial elements will tell you how much money you will need to start your business and to keep it operating until it generates enough money to pay for itself.

Although your banker will examine your entire business plan when you apply for business loans, this is the area he or she will examine most closely. This information, more than anything else, will tell the banker whether you have a clear grasp of your situation.

Your first consideration is the physical facility you will utilize. How large is the building? Where is it located? What utilities are available? Although the type of salon you want to operate will determine the type of equipment you'll need, the size of the building will determine the maximum amount of equipment you'll be able to handle. Are you renting the building or buying it? How much is the monthly rent or mortgage payment? In the case of rented facilities, don't forget to include additional rents and security deposits. Also consider the length of your lease. How long are you committed? What penalties will you incur if you break the lease? How much is the rent likely to increase when you renew the lease? What will you do if the owner doesn't want to renew your lease and you're forced to move? In the case of a building you own, don't forget property taxes and escrow payments.

You will also have to consider what it will take to make the building suitable for your use. Is there adequate electricity, heat, air conditioning, and hot water? Are the rest room facilities adequate? What will be your average monthly cost for heat, air conditioning, and electricity? How much will your water and sewer bills be? Are renovations necessary? At the very least, you'll have to wallpaper and paint. At worst, you may have to make structural changes, such as adding partitions or removing walls. Are you going to do this work yourself or hire a contractor? How long will it take to do the work? Do you risk losing income or your following while it is being done? Be realistic about your ability to do the work yourself. Estimate closely how much the work will cost, both for materials and for labor. Don't forget to allow for license and inspection fees needed for extensive renovation work. And before you start, make sure the area is zoned for the type of business you want to operate. Become familiar with the local zoning ordinances.

Don't forget about your sign. This is a very important part of your business and can be a significant one-time cost. Consider your signage requirements and get cost estimates from sign companies, then use the average figure for your planning. Also, check local ordinances for signage requirements for businesses in the area to make sure you know what is allowed and what isn't. In some cases, depending on the location, check your lease to see what kinds of signs may be prohibited.

Next, consider your capital equipment requirements. These include those pieces of machinery or apparatus necessary to perform the services you want to provide as well as equipment for the administrative aspects. This type of equipment is fixed, as for example, sinks, mirrors, and furniture, or specialized, such as facial steamers and manicure tables. It may also include items such as reception desks, computers, and display cases for retail merchandise. It generally consists of equipment that is purchased once and is amortized over a period of years.

Also consider your noncapital equipment requirements. These include items such as scissors and other implements, and consist of equipment that has a shorter life span and can be fully deducted in the purchase year as a business expense. Don't forget other significant one-time expenses, such as graphic design fees for logos, and layouts for business cards and brochures. Printing costs can be a significant start-up expense.

Using your mission statement and short-term goals as a guide, determine what and how much equipment you will need. Will you purchase or lease it? Where will you purchase it? Will you get new or used equipment? How much will it cost? Don't forget to include delivery or set-up charges. Shop around for equipment. Get the best equipment you can. Cheap equipment is no bargain. Check a number of suppliers and work with the ones who are most willing to help you. Remember, you are their customer and deserve the same consideration you give to your customers.

Supplies come next. You will need a minimum of supplies just to get started. These include consumable items such as cleansers and masks, disposable items such as disposable bonnets and cotton pads, and reusable items such as smocks and towels. Estimate your needs for consumable and disposable items for at least one month, and base your figure on the cost of those. Then add the costs for a reasonable supply of the reusable items. Shop for your suppliers of these items as carefully as you do for suppliers of the capital and noncapital equipment.

You must also allow for your staffing needs. Again, based on your mission statement and short-term goals, what is the minimum number of employees you will need to start? What type of employees will you need? Depending on the services you will offer, you may need estheticians, receptionists, electrologists, manicurists, and makeup artists. Don't forget to include yourself and any working partners who may be involved in the enterprise. How much are you going to pay these people? Where are you going to get the money to pay for their first month's work? Don't forget to include your own first month's salary requirement.

Estimated salaries are not the only expense you should consider at this point. You will also have to allow for benefits and other employee costs, such as worker's compensation and social security payments.

Also consider services you will purchase, including accounting, bookkeeping, and legal services as well as towel and laundry services. Don't forget telephone services. Get estimates from a number of suppliers to use in your planning. Add in, also, any fees you may be required to pay, such as licensing fees, fictitious name registrations, etc.

You will also have to allow some preliminary expenses for advertising and promotion. The initial campaigns will have to be ready to start shortly before you open your doors so you can begin building your business immediately. At the least, you should allow for telephone directory advertisements and local newspaper ads.

Use the figures you've established for each of these categories to develop a preliminary budget. Divide the categories into fixed expenses and one-time expenses and list them. Fixed expenses are those expenses that recur on a regular basis, such as rent, salaries, and utilities. One-time expenses are those that occur once, such as equipment, renovation costs, moving costs, etc. Total the numbers for each type of expense, then add the totals together. This will tell you how much money you will need to get your business started.

Now you should establish your time lines. How long will it take you to accomplish the various tasks necessary to start your business? List everything you have to do in the order each task must be done, then assign a tentative date to each. For example, when will you sign a lease on your facility? When will you start renovations? When will they be finished? When can you move in? When will equipment be ordered? Be delivered? When will you hire your staff? When will your advertising start? When will you open your doors for business?

This information provides you with a tentative schedule for getting your business started. It also lets you know when money will have to be spent. In addition, the time line gives you a logical sequence for getting each task accomplished and will help you keep from overlooking anything.

By this time, you've established your mission and your goals, and you've determined what you need to accomplish them. You've ascertained your needs and requirements and have set up your schedule with your time line. And, from your preliminary budget, you know how much money you need to get started. Now, you must consider where that money is going to come from.

Do you have some or all of the money you need, or will you have to borrow it? What is the source of the money you have? Is it from savings? From the sale of other assets? From other sources of income? How much of your own money are you willing or able to provide? If you have partners, how much will they provide?

How much will you have to borrow? Will you borrow from friends or family, or will you seek personal loans or second mortgage loans? Will you use credit cards or get credit from suppliers? Will you try to get a business loan from banks or finance companies? If you borrow money, how will you pay it back? What terms will you require? What will you offer as collateral?

At this point, you should develop a financial statement that lists your assets and liabilities. The statement should show any and all sources of income, as well as assets such as equity in your home, savings, stocks and bonds, etc. It should also list your personal debts, such as mortgages, credit card payments, and auto loans. Once you've done your personal financial statement, you should do an income and expense projection for your first year of operation. This information will be vital for your banker. Lending institutions can provide the funds you need, but they need to know what kind of risk you represent. Generally, the more of your own money you are able to put up, the more willing they will be to lend you the rest.

The process of building a sound, realistic business plan may seem daunting, but it is one of the most important tasks you will undertake in starting or streamlining your salon. It will make you focus on your strengths and weaknesses, and will give you an accurate estimate of the facilities, materials, people, and money you will need to get started and to maintain your business through its initial start-up pains. You will not develop your business plan overnight. It will take time and effort to accomplish. You will have to talk to a lot of people and do a lot of research. You'll also have to do much soul searching and make some hard decisions. But the time and effort you spend here will pay great dividends in the future, by well preparing you for success.

SUMMARY

The business plan is the most important document you will generate when you start your business. The exercise will make you think about what you are trying to accomplish. In addition, it will form the basis for the information you will have to supply to your bank or other financial institutions when you apply for loans.

Your business plan is the basic blueprint for your business. It enunciates your goals, your hopes and dreams, and points out how you expect to accomplish them. It is a document that is never truly finished, but one that will constantly be revised as your conditions and goals change.

There are two major segments of the business plan: the nonfinancial aspects and the financial aspects. The nonfinancial portion starts with your mission statement—a declaration of the type of business you envision. It also includes a brief biography of yourself and your partners. In essence, it is a statement of your qualifications for running the business. It lists your education, training, and experience.

The competitive situation and the demographic data also go here. Together, this information helps you determine the outside factors you will face. Next, you will characterize your potential customers. Finally, you will include a statement of your goals. They must be specific, attainable, and measurable.

The financial aspects cover the more tangible portion of the plan. Here you will examine what you need to accomplish your goals. You will consider such factors as location, equipment and supply requirements, staffing and services. Your budget and time lines will also be included. This portion will tell you how much money you will need to start the business and to keep it running and will indicate where you expect the money to come from.

It is impossible to underestimate the value of your business plan. It takes a lot of time and effort to generate, but the results you get from it are well worth it.

BUSINESS ORGANIZATION

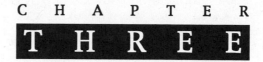

C H A P T E R
THREE

How you organize as a business can have a profound effect on your salon. The type of organization you choose affects your profits, your liability, your taxes, and your management. There are three legal forms of business organization: the sole proprietorship, the partnership, and the corporation. In addition, there are two forms of corporation: the S-corporation and the C-corporation.

Each form of organization has advantages and disadvantages. All types are valid and all work. The organization that will work best for you depends on your needs and how you want to protect yourself. Consider the pros and cons of each type carefully, then seek the advice of your accountant and your attorney.

SOLE PROPRIETORSHIP

The sole proprietorship is the simplest form of business organization and the easiest to establish. It is the legal form your business will automatically take if you are the only owner and don't choose another form of organization. As a sole proprietor, you are the single owner of your salon. You are responsible to no one but yourself. You make all the decisions and reap all the rewards, but you also take all the risks.

CHECKLIST 3-1
BUSINESS ORGANIZATION

Types of Business Organization:

1. Sole proprietorship–ownership by only one person.
    A. Advantages
        1. Simplicity–easy to form and to operate.
        2. Full ownership of profits–profits are not shared.
        3. Taxation–profits are taxed as ordinary income.
    B. Disadvantages
        1. Liability–owner has full liability; personal assets are at risk.
2. Partnership–ownership shared by one or more general or limited partners.
    A. Advantages
        1. More capital–each partner brings cash to the transaction.
        2. Taxation–profits are taxed as ordinary income.
    B. Disadvantages
        1. Liability–general partners have full liability; personal assets are at risk.
        2. Less flexibility–decisions must be made jointly.
3. C-corporation–business becomes a legal entity, chartered by the state and separate from the owners.
    A. Advantages
        1. Increased capital–owners can sell shares to raise capital.
        2. Limited liability–owners' liability is limited to the value of their ownership in the business; personal assets are not at risk.
        3. Ownership is easily transferred; stockholders can sell stock without agreement of other owners.
    B. Disadvantages
        1. Double taxation–profits are taxed at the corporate rate, then taxed as ordinary income when distributed to the owners.
        2. Difficult to set up–establishing a corporation requires a lot of time and effort.

4. S-corporation–a special type of corporation with specific limitations; combines advantages of other types of organization.
    A. Advantages
        1. Increased capital–owners can sell shares to raise capital.
        2. Limited liability–owners' liability is limited to the value of their ownership in the business; personal assets are not at risk.
        3. Ownership is easily transferred; stockholders can sell stock without agreement of other owners.
        4. Taxation–profits are taxed as ordinary income to the owners, not taxed first at the corporate rate.
    B. Disadvantages
        1. Restrictions on operation–S-corporations must meet a number of strictures to operate.
        2. Difficult to set up–establishing an S-corporation requires a lot of time and effort.

The main advantage of a sole proprietorship is its simplicity. It is a very flexible form of business. You can make decisions quickly, and you can react to changing market needs rapidly because you don't have to get agreement from anyone else. Also, you own the profits. You don't have to share them. The business doesn't pay federal income taxes on the profits. Rather, the profits are taxed as ordinary income on your personal income tax return, whether you take a salary from the business or you reinvest the proceeds in the business. By the same token, you can deduct losses from the business from other income you may have.

The main disadvantage of a sole proprietorship is liability. You are responsible for debts and judgments against the business. If the salon does not generate enough revenue to cover your bills, your creditors can attach your personal assets—your house, your car, etc. Likewise, if a client has an accident in your salon or sues you for malpractice, and your business insurance is not enough to cover the judgment, you can lose your personal belongings.

PARTNERSHIP

A partnership is formed when two or more people agree to share ownership in a business. In a general partnership, each partner is an active participant in the day-to-day operations of the business and shares in the profits on an agreed upon basis. In a limited partnership, one or more general partners operate the business and the limited partners supply capital but make no management decisions. All of the partners, however, share in the profits on an agreed upon basis. Partnerships have much the same tax advantages and liability disadvantages as sole proprietorships. They are not quite so flexible, since decisions must be made jointly.

You can form a partnership with anyone—your spouse, relatives, friends, even strangers. Once formed, however, ownership may not be readily transferred. One partner may not sell or give his or her share to someone else without the agreement of the other partners. And, contracts entered into by one general partner bind other general partners as well.

Like the sole proprietor, general partners have unlimited liability in the business. Courts can attach the personal assets of any general partner to satisfy claims by creditors or judgments against the business. Limited partners, however, are liable only up to the amount of money they have invested in the business. They can lose their investment, but not their personal assets. Limited partnerships must be registered with the state, however, to alert creditors to the liability limitations of those individuals. Also, limited partnerships are relatively expensive to set up and maintain.

Partnerships, like sole proprietorships, do not pay federal income taxes on profits. The profits are taxed as personal income to the owners, based on their share of the proceeds. They must pay taxes on the profits, even if they don't take them out of the business. Conversely, the owners may deduct business losses from other sources of income.

The federal government has very specific rules that govern partnership taxation. The partnership files Form 1065, *U. S. Partnership Return of Income.* This is an information return, not a tax return. The partnership gives each partner a Schedule K, *Partners' Shares of Income, Credits, Deductions, Etc.* The partners use the information from this document to file their individual Form 1040 tax returns. IRS

Publication 541, *Tax Information on Partnerships*, provides complete information on current IRS regulations. Your accountant will be thoroughly familiar with these regulations and procedures.

It is easy to form a partnership. All it requires is agreement among the parties involved. The agreement can be verbal, but in the best interests of the business and of the partners, there should be a written agreement that spells out all the details of the partnership, no matter how closely related or friendly the partners are. The agreement should clearly state the duties and rights of all the partners, the amount of capital each partner is to invest, the portion of the business each will own, and the share of the profits or losses each will receive. It should also include means of resolving disputes among the partners and how assets will be distributed if the business is terminated. Your attorney, in consultation with the partners, should draw up the agreement.

No matter how closely related to or friendly with your partners you are, disputes will inevitably arise. A well-thought-out written agreement will make those disputes easier to settle and will prevent undue stress on the business. Without a written agreement, the courts will likely decide that the partnership was equal, when that may never have been intended. An oral agreement will have practically no weight in court or in arbitration.

CORPORATION

A corporation is a legal body, sanctioned by the state in which it is registered. Unlike a proprietorship or partnership, a corporation exists as a legal entity, separate from its owners. Whereas a proprietorship or partnership dissolves on the death of the proprietor or one of the partners, the corporation continues even after the death of the individual owners. It is more complicated to set up than the other forms of organization, and its operation is more tightly controlled by various government bodies.

The major advantage of a corporation is limited liability on the part of the owners. Unlike proprietors or general partners, stockholders in a corporation cannot lose their personal assets to settle creditor claims or judgments against the business. They can only lose what they have invested in the corporation. Keep in mind, however, that if you incorporate your salon, because of its small size, bankers and suppliers may still require you to use your personal assets as collateral. In this case, you haven't lessened your liability to major financial creditors, but your personal assets are protected from liability claims and lawsuits.

Another advantage of the corporation is that ownership is easily transferred. Ownership is in the form of shares of stock. All owners, i.e. stockholders, have a vote in the operation of the company in proportion to the amount of stock they hold. Any stockholder can sell his or her stock in the corporation to someone else without the agreement of the other stockholders.

It is normally easier to raise capital in a corporation. Ownership of stock is generally more attractive to investors than limited investment in partnerships because of the greater security and ease of ownership transfer. However, if you offer stock to the public, you will have to register with and meet all the requirements of the Securities and Exchange Commission.

The disadvantage of a C-corporation, the standard form of incorporation, is in double taxation. Profits from the corporation are taxed at the corporate tax rate. When the profits are distributed to the stockholders as dividends, they are taxed again as personal income. Losses incurred by the corporation cannot be deducted from the stockholders' gains from other income. If the stockholders draw salaries from the company, however, those salaries are deducted from the operating expense of the corporation and are not included as profits for tax purposes. The salaries are taxed as personal income for the stockholders.

For tax purposes, stockholders who work for the corporation are considered employees of the corporation and can draw salaries. Proprietors or partners, on the other hand, are not considered employees and cannot draw salaries. They can only share in the profits.

Profits from an S-corporation are taxed differently. An S-corporation is a form of organization that combines the advantages of partnerships with corporations, giving the owners the limited liability advantages of a corporation and the tax advantages of a partnership. S-corporations do not pay income taxes on profits. Instead, the profits are taxed as ordinary income to the owners, much as they are in a partnership. However, the tax implications are complicated, so you should consult with your accountant before opting for this form of business organization. Under current tax laws, S-corporations have lost many of their advantages in terms of health care deductions and other benefits.

S-corporations have a number of requisites that C-corporations do not have. For example, ownership must be limited to thirty-five or fewer stockholders and there may be restrictions on transfer of ownership. All stockholders must be U. S. citizens or residents, and you can offer only one class of stock. If you violate any of the strictures that govern S-corporations, you can easily lose the special status and revert to a C-corporation.

Whether S- or C-, a corporation is established by registering articles of incorporation with the state in which you wish to incorporate. This does not have to be the state in which you will operate. Some states have laws that are more favorable to corporations than other states. If you choose a state other than your own, however, you will need a registered agent and a mailing address in that state to receive legal documents. If you incorporate in the state in which you operate, either you or your attorney may serve as the agent. The mailing address can be the business address.

In addition, you will need written bylaws, which detail the operation of the company, and you will have to establish a board of directors, who will elect corporate officers. These procedures are straightforward and not complicated; however, there are many legal and tax implications involved. If you choose the corporate form of organization for your business, you should work closely with your attorney and your accountant.

BUYING AN ESTABLISHED SALON

Once you've decided to open your own skin and body care salon, you can either start a new business or purchase an existing business. There are advantages and disadvantages to both. If you start a new business, you can tailor it to meet your exact needs and will not inherit a previous owner's problems. But you will have to build the business from nothing, and it may take you some time to get established and start to earn a profit.

On the other hand, if you buy an existing business, you may be able to move right into a profit-making concern. You might have an already established clientele to work with. And you will most likely

CHECKLIST 3-2
BUYING AN ESTABLISHED SALON

STEP 1: Finding the salon

1. Classified ads
2. Business brokers
3. Real estate agents
4. Word of mouth

STEP 2: Investigation

1. History of the salon
2. Reasons the owner is selling
3. Examination of owner's books and records
4. Legal audit

STEP 3: Evaluation

1. Facilities and location suitable for needs
2. Area demographics
3. Renovations needed

STEP 4: Negotiation

1. Value of physical facilities
2. Value of customer list
3. Goodwill
4. Covenant not to compete
5. Employee retention
6. Offer

keep some experienced employees. Your start-up concerns will be minimized, but you might have to offer services you're not comfortable with or be limited in the services you can offer by the existing facilities. Or, if you're not careful, you might inherit the previous owner's problems.

Whether you start from the beginning or purchase an established salon, the same principles of business apply. You will still have to follow sound business practices and think every step through. If you decide to purchase an established business, there are a number of extra considerations. Where do you find a suitable salon for sale? Just what are you buying? How do you determine its worth? How do you negotiate the sale? Buying an existing salon can be a good way to get into your own business, but there are a lot of pitfalls. So beware. Pay attention to what you're doing. Get all the advice you can, but get enough information to make the decision. Involve your attorney and accountant from the beginning. You are looking into an endeavor that will cost you thousands of dollars. Don't begrudge spending a few hundred to get expert help. But remember, no matter how much advice you get and how expert that advice is, you are still the one responsible for making the choice.

How do you find a salon that is for sale? There are a number of ways. The classified ads in the newspapers list businesses for sale. You might also go to business brokers. Business brokers operate much like real estate brokers. They act as agents for people who want to sell their businesses, maintain lists of sales opportunities, and have networks among other brokers to widen the search. Real estate agents may also be a good source for finding a business for sale, especially if the property on which it is located is for sale also. Remember, however, that brokers represent the seller and have a vested interest in making the sale. If you have a specific area in mind, you could canvass other salons in that general area and ask owners or employees if they know of any salons for sale.

Once you have found a salon, investigate it thoroughly. How long has it been in operation? If it doesn't have much of a history, beware. There may be significant problems if a business is less than two years old and is up for sale. This, in itself, doesn't mean that the salon is not a worthwhile purchase, but it should spur you to do some additional checking.

Find out why the owner is selling the salon. Is he or she retiring? Moving to another location? Selling because of illness or because he or she is just tired of the business? Or is the business for sale because it is not profitable? Does the owner know that there are plans to build a new shopping mall around the corner, which will destroy the business? There are many motives for selling a business. Some are good; others are not. It's up to you to find out the reason—the real reason—the salon that interests you is for sale. Ask the owner. Don't be afraid to ask hard, even personal questions. It is your right and is for your protection.

Thoroughly evaluate the salon according to your needs and requirements. The same location parameters apply whether you're starting a new salon or purchasing an existing salon. Is the location adequate? What is the neighborhood like? Do the people you want to service live or work in the vicinity? What other businesses operate in the area? How much possible competition is in the area? Walk around the neighborhood. Talk to other business owners. Ask about the level and quality of business in the area, and ask them specifically how the salon seems to be doing. Also, ask if there is anything planned that may affect business in the area. For example, is there a new shopping center planned that will take traffic away from the salon? Are properties being condemned because a new highway is going to be built through the neighborhood? Is the zoning up for review?

Suppose everything so far meets with your satisfaction. The salon looks promising and you think you can be successful with it. How do you determine what it is worth? The owner will have an asking price, but that does not mean it's the price you have to pay. The value of the business depends on a number of factors. When you buy an existing business, all you can purchase are the tangible assets—the fixtures, equipment, products, etc.—and intangibles such as goodwill and covenant not to compete. You cannot purchase customers. There is no guarantee that they will want to do business with you. The same holds true for employees. There's no guarantee that estheticians and other employees will want to work for you.

So concentrate on the tangible assets. First, the facilities. Is the building for sale or does the owner have a lease? If the building is for sale, have it appraised by a registered real estate appraiser. If it is rented, talk to the building's owner or agent. Make sure he or she will extend the existing lease or give you a new one. The salon owner's lease may not allow for transfers. Also, make sure that you can get a lease for a sufficient length of time to make it worthwhile, generally three to five years, and negotiate the rent before you buy the salon.

It is probably more prudent to rent rather than buy the real estate. You want your dollars invested in the salon business, not the real estate business. Remember, if you must buy the real estate to purchase the business, you are really buying two separate things—the salon business and the building. Evaluate these separately and individually. If the seller owns the building, you may be able to arrange a lease with a buy-out option.

Whether the building is for sale or rent, examine it carefully. Make sure the facilities are adequate. Have it inspected by code authorities to be sure it meets all code requirements for the locality. Is there adequate electrical power? Do you have enough hot water? Is the heating and air conditioning system in good repair? Is there adequate ventilation? Is the lighting sufficient? Is the roof in good condition? Are the rest room facilities adequate? Are there any repairs or alterations that you will have to make before you take over the business? Is there enough room for expansion? Or is there too much room for you to use? Are the floors in good condition? Will you have to redecorate? To what extent? Who is responsible for repairs to the building, you or the owner? What restrictions on signage are there? Are there any legal or contractual constraints on how you conduct the business, as to the services you can offer or the hours you can operate, for example? Is there anything about the structure that might hinder your efforts?

When you are thoroughly satisfied with the suitability of the premises, concentrate on the equipment and fixtures. Get a complete list, in writing, of the equipment the owner is selling. Ask yourself the same hard questions. Is the equipment suitable for your use? Does the style of the equipment meet your standards for decor? Is it in good condition, or must it be refurbished? Is it obsolete or does it reflect current technology? Will you have to add any new equipment? Is there equipment you don't want? Determine which pieces of equipment you will use and which pieces you won't. Then make a written list of your own, including only what interests you and meets your needs. This will be one of your negotiating points.

Get an approximate valuation of the equipment you want. You should have some idea of what it is worth from your own experience and study. In addition, you can get help from manufacturers and wholesalers. You're looking for a figure that provides the value of the equipment as it stands. Keep in mind that it is used, not new, and even only one-year-old equipment is frequently worth half its original cost. You do not want to consider what it would cost to replace the used equipment with new. You need to know the actual value, not the replacement value, which would be a far higher figure. The idea is to assign a dollar value to the equipment package. This will be one of the major points to consider in determining a fair price for the salon.

Go through the same procedures with supplies and retail products. Get a complete inventory. Find out how old the materials are, either from expiration dates on the packaging or from receipts. Determine which materials you want and which you don't want. Then figure how much they cost the owner. This cost will be higher than you should pay. Remember, you can buy all new, fresh products for approximately the same dollar amount the owner paid for the products that he or she may have had sitting on shelves for some time. Depending on the age and condition of the products, deduct from 10 to 50 percent of the owner's costs as your value. Your accountant will help you determine a reasonable percentage.

Add the value of the equipment and the supplies. (If you are purchasing the building, add that value as well.) This will give you a total value for the physical assets of the salon. Don't pay more for the assets than you would pay to buy all new equipment and supplies. You should pay less.

Placing a value on the intangible assets of the business is more difficult and more subject to interpretation. Here, you have to determine what goodwill is worth. Goodwill, as business custom defines it, is the regard a business has beyond the value of its goods and services. It is an intangible assessment of the profit potential of the business beyond what would normally be expected from a business of its kind. For example, if salons in the area can be expected to generate revenues of $100,000 per year and the salon you are interested in purchasing has yearly revenues of $115,000, the goodwill can be estimated at $15,000. Your accountant should be able to estimate the goodwill of the salon.

In many ways, goodwill is a measure of the success of the business. You can verify that success by thoroughly examining the records. Have your accountant audit the financial records of the salon for at least the last two to three years, and longer if the audit uncovers anything that looks suspicious. This includes all ledgers, journals, and financial statements. Be wary here. Owners have been known to alter books. Sometimes an owner will intimate to you that the books are only for the government and don't reflect the true revenues of the salon. No matter what the owner tells you, the only figures you should consider are those you see in the records. If the owner admits to cheating the government out of taxes, what makes you think he or she won't lie to you? Before you put up any money, look at the tax returns for at least the past three years. They may not agree with the books.

Don't limit your examination to the financial records. Look at the appointment books and other customer records for the last year or two, as well. Do the customer records verify the figures in the financial records? Has the customer flow through the salon been sufficient to generate the amount of income the ledgers show? If the appointment calendar shows that an average of ten clients a week come to the salon, but the books show weekly revenues of $5,000, there may be a discrepancy. Also check supply purchase records. Is the volume of supplies purchased consistent with the customer flow? If the records indicate that five hundred customers came through in a month, but the owner only bought two bottles of cleanser, you may have a problem. Let your own experience be a guide. If the owner agrees, spend a few days or a week working in the salon to get a feel for the traffic. This will also give you an indication of the level of work done in the salon and the type of customers that come in.

Generally, the smaller the business, the less the value of goodwill. Service businesses such as beauty salons, where the business depends on the skill of the cosmetologists, have little or no goodwill. It is the amount you will pay for the business that exceeds the value of the tangible assets and is a negotiable factor in your dealings with the owner or broker. You want to pay as little as possible for goodwill.

The other intangible asset you want to negotiate is a covenant not to compete. This means you want an agreement, as part of the terms of sale, that the previous owner will not open or work in another salon within a specified area for a specified time. An example would be an agreement that prevents the owner from opening a salon within a ten-mile radius for a period of three years. Such agreements are enforceable as long as they are reasonable. You cannot prevent someone from making a living, but you can give yourself some breathing room. Your attorney will be able to advise you on this aspect of the agreement.

Like goodwill, a covenant not to compete has a negotiable value. You should expect to pay something for the agreement. For tax purposes, the amount you pay for goodwill is not deductible as an expense. The amount you pay for the covenant not to compete, however, like the tangible assets you purchase, is deductible as depreciation.

Noncompete payments are a good way of paying for the business over time. For example, if the business is worth $100,000, you might offer $70,000 plus $10,000 per year noncompete for three years.

While your accountant is auditing the books, have your attorney conduct a legal audit. He or she will make sure there are no outstanding liabilities, such as debts or malpractice suits, hanging over the salon. If you purchase a salon with such liabilities, you may be responsible for paying them. There are some liabilities you may have to assume. If the owner owes money for recently purchased equipment, for example, you might take over the payments as part of the deal. In such a case, however, the amount of those liabilities will be deducted from the assets.

Even if you buy only assets, be aware that you can get stuck with liabilities. For example, if the seller didn't pay back phone bills or Yellow Pages charges, the phone company will revoke your number. So all your ads and Yellow Page work will go for nothing. Or, for instance, you may not owe for past due electric, water and sewer bills, but utilities will turn off your power and water while you sort out who's responsible for past debts. One way to solve this is to hold back money from the sales transaction and put it into escrow. The seller gets the money with interest after a year if there are no surprise debts.

Determine the salon's organization type. If it is a sole proprietorship, the owner will have the authority to sell the business. If it is a partnership, make sure all the partners agree to the terms of the sale. If the salon is incorporated, you must decide whether you are buying the assets or the owners' stock. If you buy the stock, the corporation continues to exist as a legal entity and you will operate under the corporate charter. If you buy the assets, however, the corporation ceases to exist, and you will create a new company that you may organize in any form you wish. If the salon is a franchise operation, you may also have to negotiate with the franchisor, who will most likely have a voice in any new ownership of the salon.

Once you have completed your examination of the business and everything meets your standards, you can open negotiations with the owner. Add the figures for the tangible and intangible assets to determine a dollar value of the business. Also, decide how much the business is worth to you. In other words, how much do you want the business? This will determine your opening offer. The owner will probably return with a counteroffer. This is a normal part of business negotiation, so don't be upset with the give and take. Remember, in any negotiations, as long as both parties are negotiating in good faith, a good deal is one that satisfies the needs of both sides.

Be firm in the negotiations, but be fair. Know how far you are willing to go and don't go past that point, even if it means walking away from the salon. Don't get emotionally involved with the salon. No matter how much you may want to buy it, make the deal with your brain, not your heart. Don't let your desire outrun your common sense.

FRANCHISE OPERATIONS

Another method of acquiring a salon is through the purchase of a franchise. A franchise is a type of licensing arrangement in which, for certain specified fees, royalties, and service charges, you buy into a network of businesses and acquire the rights to use the franchisor's trademarks, services, and products, and to trade on the franchisor's reputation and goodwill, built up through the other franchisees.

Like any form of business organization, franchising has both advantages and disadvantages. As a salon franchisee, you are an independent business person, affiliated with other salon franchisees of that same chain. You get the advantage of combined economic leverage, technical and managerial assistance, and regional or national advertising and promotion that you wouldn't have as a totally independent salon owner.

The disadvantage of a franchise is the loss of a good measure of independence. Whether you want one or not, you have a partner, and that partner will exercise significant control over how you conduct the business. The franchisor may require you to offer specific services, to operate certain hours, and to purchase equipment and supplies from a limited number of suppliers. In addition, the royalty payments and service fees may be particularly onerous. These payments are generally based on gross receipts (that is, revenues before deducting expenses) and must be paid whether or not you're left with a profit.

Franchises are regulated by the Federal Trade Commission's Disclosure Rule, which requires franchisors to divulge all pertinent information about the franchise. The rule requires current and accurate information on twenty subjects, including the history and operation of the franchisor, the obligations of the franchisee, fees and costs needed, and the services and property the franchisee receives for those fees and costs. Franchisor history includes the length of time the company has been in business, the experience it has in the field, the experience of directors and executives, and legal history, including past and present lawsuits against the company. The franchisor must also provide financial statements for the company and statistical information about the identity, number, and locations of other franchisees.

Franchisee obligations include information about fees, restrictions on the conduct of the business, with whom the franchisee may do business, and what products and equipment the franchisee must purchase from the franchisor. The disclosure must specify the length of the franchise term and renewal options and spell out termination requirements. Also included is information about training, advertising and promotion, and celebrity involvement.

If the franchisor makes any claims about potential profit, additional disclosures are required. In addition to the federal laws, many states have their own regulations governing franchises.

If you decide to pursue a franchise opportunity, don't rely solely on the disclosure statement. Conduct your own investigation and get your accountant and attorney involved in the process. Talk to other franchisees, and don't limit your conversations to the ones recommended by the franchisor. Examine the track record of the franchisor. How long has the company been in business? How many franchisees are there? Does the franchisor also operate company stores that may compete with the franchisees? How does the company get most of its income—from the franchise fees up front, or from the ongoing royalties and service fees? What kind of support does the franchisor give? Do they offer financial assistance? Do they provide locations or assist in finding a location? What kinds of training programs are available? What rules and restrictions are contained in the franchise agreement? Do you have to buy goods and services from the franchisor, or can you shop on your own? What records do you have to keep? What kind of reporting is required? How exclusive is the territory they offer? Will you have to compete with their other franchisees in your area?

Look at every aspect of the franchise agreement. Be objective and be thorough. Take the time to make a reasoned decision based on facts. Let your attorney examine the agreement, and let your accountant examine the financial statements.

Shop for the franchise just as you would for any other commodity. In the beauty industry, there are more than thirty franchisors offering a variety of hair, skin, nail, and body services. The franchise and set-up fees vary from a low of $25,000 to a high of $176,000. The average cost for buying a franchise and opening the salon is $60,000 to $80,000. Some of the money must come from your own rather than from borrowed funds.

Some franchisors are large, with more than two thousand franchisees; others are small, with two or three. Some have been in business for more than thirty years, some for only one or two years. Most offer training in salon operation and management techniques. Most do not offer financial assistance, but some will help you get the help you need. A few will provide you with a location as part of the fee; most will not. You will have to find your own location. Many of the salons you see in large malls and shopping centers are franchise operations.

Many franchisors require you to purchase their own private label products and specify the equipment you must purchase. Many operate their own company stores in addition to the franchises they sell. Some of these companies have more company stores than franchisees.

Franchising can be a way to open a salon and get into business quickly with relatively limited resources. It can also be a very perilous process, so be careful. If you decide to take this path, get the prospectuses from each of the franchisors that interest you and compare them. Choose the one that gives you the best opportunity. But, under any circumstances, investigate thoroughly before you invest your money.

SUMMARY

You may organize your business in one of three forms. The simplest is the sole proprietorship, in which you are the only owner. The profits you make as a sole proprietor are taxed as ordinary income. However, you bear full liability for judgments against the business.

In a partnership, you share ownership and profits with one or more partners, who may be either general partners or limited partners. General partners are active participants in the business; limited partners supply capital but do not operate the business. The tax advantages are the same as for a sole proprietorship, as are the liability disadvantages.

A corporation is a legal entity, separate from the stockholders. The advantage of incorporating is that liability is limited to the company and not to the personal assets of the owners. In a C-corporation, the standard form, the disadvantage is in double taxation. The C-corporation pays taxes on profits, and the owners pay taxes on those profits when they take them out as dividends. In an S-corporation, profits are taxed as ordinary income to the owners.

There are also three ways to get into business. You can start a salon from nothing, purchase an existing salon, or buy a franchise. If you start from nothing, you can build the business exactly the way you want, but you start without a continuing base of operations. If you buy a salon, you start with an established business, but you run the risk of inheriting the previous owner's problems. If you buy a franchise, you are getting, in effect, a license to use the franchisor's name and products, and can gain the advantages of an existing network of experience. However, you will not be independent. You must follow the rules and procedures established by the franchisor.

Whether you buy an existing salon or a franchise, it is vital that you thoroughly investigate all aspects of the deal. Learn all you can about either, then exercise caution.

ESTHETICS SERVICES

C H A P T E R
FOUR

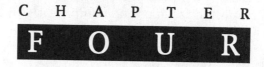

The type of salon you operate will depend on the services you want to offer and the clientele you want to serve. The services can be as varied or as specific as you desire and, to a large extent, will reflect your ability and your interests. You may decide you want to offer a full range of skin and body care services, or you may decide you want to offer only basic skin care services.

Similarly, you can define the clientele you want to service as widely or narrowly as you wish. Establish a profile of your primary intended clients. Do you wish to perform your services on women only? On men only? On children? Or do you expect to service any combination of these? What age range do you wish to service? The services you offer and the clientele you offer them to are interrelated, so you must consider both when you make your decisions. For example, you would probably not offer full body waxing services if your intended customers were primarily men.

Your decision will also be determined, in part, by the demographics and needs of the area in which you locate. Your preliminary examinations of your intended area of operation should have revealed how many and what type of people who will make up your customer base live and work there. And your surveys of other salons in the area, along with talking to as many people as you could, should have given you a good idea of what skin and body care services those

47

people want and which services you can profitably offer. Remember, your object is to make a profit. It makes no sense to spend the money for equipment, facilities, and training to offer a service you can't sell. You are better served by using that money, time, and energy to establish popular services that will be profitable.

Each type of skin and body care salon has its own set of needs with respect to facilities and equipment. And each type has its own requirements for talent, training, and cost to establish and operate. So, base your decision on your personality, interests, ability, and pocketbook. Whichever type of salon you choose to operate, however, will have to generate a rate of return to fit the lifestyle you want. That means you may have to offer services that don't particularly interest you to generate sales of the services that do. So, choose wisely and judiciously. Offer as many different services as you are comfortable with. Keep in mind that it is not necessary to offer every service that interests you at the beginning. You can add more services as your business grows. Concentrate on your basic, income-producing services first. Regardless of which combinations of services you choose to offer, any service you give in your salon should either make a profit or lead to sales of other, more profitable services.

SALON SERVICES

Today's skin and body care salons offer an amazing variety of services, from the simple and traditional, such as facials and body waxing, to the esoteric, such as body wraps and spa treatments. All of these services are designed to enhance the clients' appearance, and in some cases, help them to achieve a healthier lifestyle.

All services, however, must be limited to application on the exterior of the head, hands, feet, or body. No service given may involve the internal application of any implement or substance. No service may be sold for anything more than improvement of appearance, even if there may be some health-giving aspect to the service. Remember always, a skin care salon is not a medical facility and may undertake no operation that impinges on medical services.

Cosmetology, of which esthetics is a branch, is a highly regulated profession. Most of the services offered may be given only by a properly licensed practitioner in a duly licensed salon. In virtually all states, staff members must possess valid licenses. Just about the only employees exempt from this stricture are receptionists. License requirements vary somewhat from state to state, so check with your state licensing board for the latest regulations.

There are five general categories of skin care salon services: those for skin and body care, those for hair removal, those for makeup application and cosmetics, those for nails, and retail sales. Each service in each category has its own special requirements with respect to training, licensing, and equipment and supplies needed. Keep in mind, however, that some equipment may be used for more than one type of service.

CHECKLIST 4-1
ESTHETICS SERVICES

There are five categories of services:

1. Skin and Body Care Services
   A. Facials
   B. Body Massage
   C. Wraps and Packs
   D. Hydrotherapy Treatments
2. Hair Removal Services
3. Makeup Services
   A. Application of Cosmetics
   B. Consultation
   C. Color Analyses
   D. Ear Piercing
4. Nail Services
   A. Manicures
   B. Pedicures
   C. Nail Wrapping
   D. Sculptured Nail Application
   E. Artificial Nail Application
   F. Nail Painting
   G. Nail Tipping
5. Retail Sales

Equipment may be categorized as capital and noncapital equipment. Capital equipment has a long life span and is depreciated over a period of years. It includes fixtures such as mirrors, facial chairs, skin care machinery, and display cases. Noncapital equipment has a relatively short life span and is written off in the year it is purchased. This includes tools such as scissors and Wood's lamps.

Supplies may be categorized as reusable, disposable, and expendable. Reusable supplies are items that are used repeatedly and include towels and smocks. Disposable items are those that are used once and discarded and include cotton pads and disposable bonnets. Expendable supplies are those that are consumed during use and include masks, cleansers, toners, etc.

The division of equipment and supplies into such specific categories may seem moot, but they are important distinctions. Thinking of these items in these terms will force you to think more like a business person and will enable you to keep track of your expenses and to allocate charges more accurately. It will also help when you fill out your tax returns.

Don't stint on equipment or supplies. Get the best you can afford. Don't be afraid of buying used equipment as long as it is in good condition. Top-quality equipment looks more professional, works more efficiently, and lasts longer than cheap equipment. Your equipment quality will tell your prospective clients a lot about the quality of your services. In the beginning, at least, get only what you need. Idle equipment costs money. You want to maximize the use of the equipment you have. Keep it working for you, not against you. You can always add more later, when business warrants it. The business aspects of purchasing or leasing equipment are covered in chapter 11.

SKIN AND BODY CARE SERVICES

Over the past few years, skin care and body services have undergone tremendous growth. They are popular among both men and women and are a profitable source of revenue, although they require considerable capital equipment and supplies as well as special training. Many of these services complement each other and may be offered in various combinations. These must be performed by properly licensed cosmetologists.

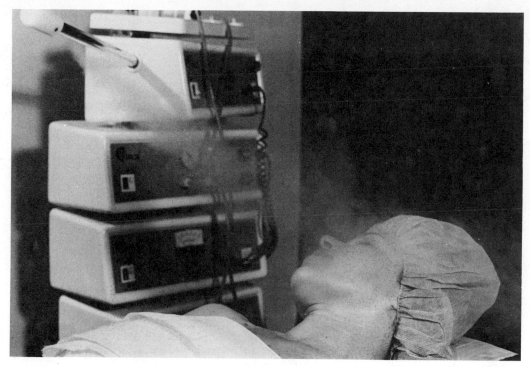

FIGURE 4-1 Facial treatment

Facials

The facial is the cornerstone of skin care in the salon (Figure 4-1). It is the most widely offered of the skin care services and has significant profit potential. Facials may be offered to men as well as women. Although women receive most of the facial services, men represent a largely untapped potential customer base.

Facials require a considerable amount of equipment to perform properly. Although it is possible to give facials without it, to establish the professional image you will need to succeed, you must have the proper equipment. Your clients will expect no less, and they deserve no less.

Facials may be given by a licensed cosmetologist or esthetician. Most beauty schools cover facials in at least a rudimentary fashion in the normal hair dressing curriculum. Many schools also offer specific training in esthetics. In addition, advanced training is available through courses offered by the manufacturers of equipment and supplies.

EQUIPMENT   The basic piece of capital equipment for facials is the reclining padded facial chair, which may be the same chair used for waxing. The other essentials are a magnifying lamp and a padded stool or chair for the esthetician. Theoretically, facials may be given without any other equipment. In practice, however, much more specialized equipment is needed. This includes steamers, galvanic current machines, high-frequency machines, rotary brush machines, vacuum/spray machines, dry sanitizers, and Wood's lamps. Optional capital equipment may include paraffin baths, infrared lamps, and electric pulverizators.

Noncapital equipment includes a variety of brushes for the rotary brush machine, different size ventouses for the vacuum/spray machine, spray bottles, smocks, and gowns. Supplies include cotton, viscose sponges, spatulas, disposable head covers, various types of cleansers, toners, astringents, masks, oils, and treatment products.

Body Massage

Various forms of theraputic massage are becoming increasingly popular and can be profitable services to offer, either in specialized massage salons or in other types of salons as adjuncts to facials and other skin care services (Figure 4-2). The services are applicable to both men and women.

Training and licensing requirements vary from state to state. In most states, licensed estheticians and cosmetologists may give basic facial massages and massages to the hands and feet. Full body massage, however, often requires a special license as a massage therapist. Check your state laws before offering massage services. The procedures do require considerable training and practice. Basic training in massage of the face, hands, and feet is normally given as part of the curriculum for estheticians and cosmetologists. Training in the various full-body massage techniques is available from special schools.

EQUIPMENT   The most important piece of capital equipment is a top-quality padded massage table. Additional capital equipment includes a chair or stool for the massage therapist, heat and ultraviolet

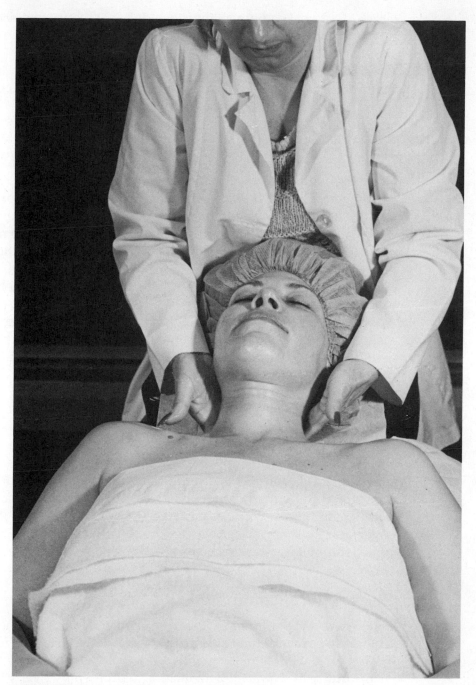

FIGURE 4-2 Body massage treatment

lamps. Optional equipment may include high-frequency machines and galvanic current machines (the same as used in facials). You should also have shower facilities available.

Noncapital equipment includes dressing gowns or smocks, oral thermometers, sheets, and blankets. Supplies include towels, cotton, spatulas, and a variety of massage creams and oils.

Wraps and Packs

Body wraps and various packs are used for a variety of cellulite, cleansing, and water retention treatments in spas and salons. These treatments, of interest primarily to women, are gaining in popularity and can be profitable adjuncts to a salon that specializes in skin and body care. In essence, these services eliminate or redistribute retained body water or fat cells to achieve a temporary slimming and tightening effect. Some of the services also stimulate and balance certain body systems such as the lymphatic and circulatory systems and help cleanse impurities from the body.

The services may be given by licensed estheticians and cosmetologists. Training in the application and use of body wraps and packs is included in most curriculums for estheticians. Additional training is offered by manufacturers of equipment and products.

EQUIPMENT   The capital equipment requirements for wraps and packs is much the same as for facials and massage. Most important are a padded reclining facial chair or massage table, a chair or stool for the facialist, and heat lamps. Steamers, rotary brush machines, and other electrical equipment used for facials may also be included. Noncapital equipment includes blankets, sheets, spatulas, spray bottles, and timers. Supplies include towels, cotton, disposable head covers, plastic wrap, elastic bandages, and various algae and mud pack compounds, cleansing creams, astringents, and treatment creams.

Hydrotherapy Treatments

Like wraps and packs, hydrotherapy treatments are highly specialized services for cleansing and balancing internal body systems (Figure 4-3). Thalassotherapy treatments utilize sea water. Balneotherapy treatments utilize fresh water. Both include hydrotherapy tubs, whirlpool baths, hot tubs, and Scotch hose treatment. These services, again of

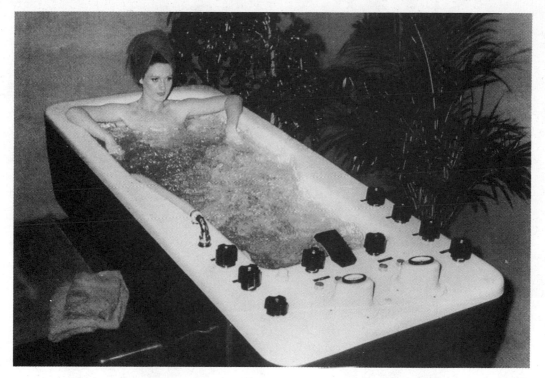

FIGURE 4-3 Hydrotherapy treatment

interest mostly to women, are profitable for spas and skin care salons, but require very expensive capital equipment and facilities. State licensing requirements vary, but these treatments may usually be given by licensed estheticians, physical therapists, and massage therapists, although more specialized training in the proper use of these devices is required.

EQUIPMENT   Capital equipment includes hydrotherapy tubs, whirlpool baths, hot tubs and high pressure hose systems, high capacity hot water systems, and shower facilities. Some areas may require water softening units, as well. Noncapital equipment includes brushes, sheets, gowns, and robes. Supplies include towels, mineral bath preparations, bath oils, and lotions, as well as a variety of mud and algae preparations.

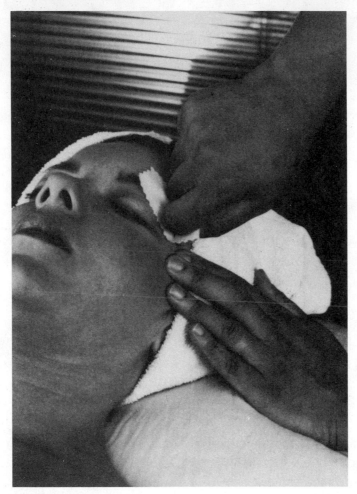

FIGURE 4-4 Hair removal treatment

HAIR REMOVAL SERVICES

The removal of excess or unwanted body and facial hair is a growing
area for the modern salon (Figure 4-4). Offered as an adjunct to other
services, or offered as a specialty, this can be profitable and can bring
considerable new and repeat business to your operation. There are
four basic hair removal methods—shaving, chemical depilation,
waxing, and electrolysis. Generally, only waxing and electrolysis are
offered as skin care salon services.

Waxing

Waxing is a relatively simple and efficient method for temporarily removing hair from the face and body. It requires a minimum of equipment and is relatively inexpensive for the client, yet provides a good source of revenue. It can be offered to both men and women, although women require the service more often than men. The service may be performed by a licensed cosmetologist or esthetician. Basic training in waxing techniques are covered in many beauty school curriculums. Additional on-the-job training may be advisable to build proficiency.

EQUIPMENT Capital equipment includes padded, reclining treatment chairs or padded tables and thermostatically controlled heaters to melt and hold the wax at a constant temperature. Other equipment includes tweezers, scissors, smocks, and drapes. Supplies include hair removal wax, muslin strips, wooden spatulas, skin cleansing creams and astringents, cotton, rolls of paper like those used on physicians' examining tables to protect the equipment, and antiseptic lotions.

Electrolysis

Electrolysis, the only method of removing hair permanently, is fairly expensive to establish but is highly profitable. Most salons that offer electrolysis specialize in the service, but it can be offered with other services. It is a specially good fit with other skin care services and is popular among both men and women. Electrolysis is a highly skilled specialty and, in most states, requires a separate electrologist license. A number of schools offer electrology curriculums leading to the license. Practice is also required to gain proficiency.

EQUIPMENT Capital equipment includes conventional needle or tweezer radio frequency epilators or galvanic epilators, padded reclining treatment chairs, electrologists' stools, equipment tables, sterilizers, magnifying lamps, and mirrors. Other equipment includes a supply of electrolysis needles, tweezers, scissors, smocks, and drapes. Supplies include towels, cotton, tissues, eye shields, skin cleansing creams, astringents, and antiseptic lotions.

MAKEUP AND COSMETICS APPLICATION SERVICES

Makeup and cosmetics application and consultation services are widely popular (Figure 4-5). Offered as an adjunct to skin care services, or alone as a specialty, they can be very profitable among

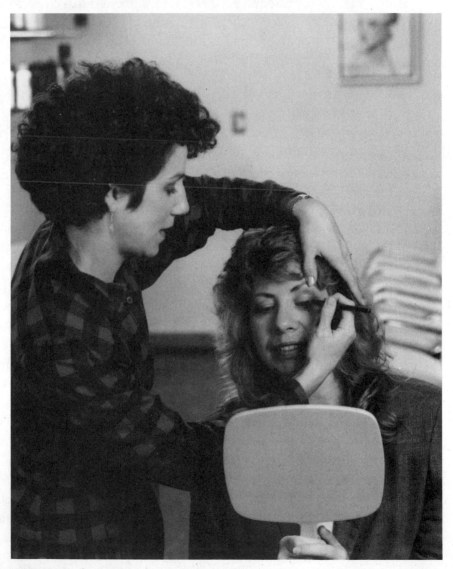

FIGURE 4-5 Makeup application

female clients. Compared with some other salon services, they are relatively inexpensive to offer and require minimal capital equipment, although supply outlays may be large. The services, which may range from offering advice to women on what makeup to use and how to apply it to the application of corrective makeup to cover blemishes to ear piercing, can be given by a licensed cosmetologist or esthetician. Basic training in makeup use and application techniques is part of many beauty school curriculums. Additional training is available through cosmetics manufacturers and wholesalers.

EQUIPMENT   Capital equipment includes a makeup stand or counter, a large mirror ringed with lights that can be adjusted to simulate daylight and evening lighting conditions, and a hydraulic chair, such as the type used for hair services. Noncapital equipment includes a variety of makeup brushes, viscose sponges, hand mirrors, sanitizers, smocks, and capes. Supplies include quantities of foundations, corrective makeup, blushes, eye shadows, powders, lipsticks, mascaras, false eyelashes, cotton, disposable head covers, and spatulas.

NAIL SERVICES

Nail services are very popular and profitable and can be offered in conjunction with skin care services (Figure 4-6). Although more popular among women, many men get basic manicures. Advanced nail techniques are usually offered to women only.

It is also possible to offer only nail services, including manicures and pedicures. Many successful salons of this type are in operation. In addition to basic manicure services, you might also offer advanced services such as nail wrapping, sculptured nails, artificial nail application, nail painting, and nail tipping.

Most states require that the practitioner hold either a manicurist license or a cosmetology license. Manicuring is covered as part of the standard cosmetology curriculum or is offered as a separate course in most beauty schools, and additional training in nail structure and the recognition of nail disorders is advisable. Specialized training in advanced manicuring techniques is available through special classes offered by many suppliers.

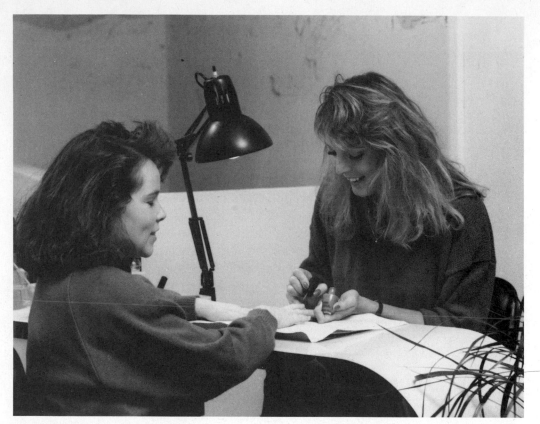

FIGURE 4-6 Manicuring

EQUIPMENT   Capital equipment for manicuring includes manicure tables, adjustable lamps, padded chairs for the clients, and padded stools or chairs for the manicurist. Other equipment includes supply trays, finger bowls, heaters for oil, wet sanitizers, and assorted containers, as well as nail files, cuticle pushers, cuticle scissors or nippers, nail brushes, nail buffers, tweezers, small application brushes and spatulas. Supplies include towels, cotton, orangewood sticks, and emery boards. Also included in the supply list are nail cleansers, polish removers, cuticle oils and creams, cuticle removers, nail bleaches and whiteners, assorted nail polishes, thinners, base coats, top coats, nail hardeners, nail dryers, hand creams and lotions, antiseptics, tissues, alcohol, mending silk or tissue, adhesives, and assorted artificial nails.

For sculptured nail application add nail forms, measuring spoons, acrylic nippers, mixing bowls, and application brushes. An optional piece of capital equipment for sculptured nails is a special ultraviolet light source for curing the acrylic resins.

The equipment required for offering pedicures is much the same as for manicures. In addition, you will need a low stool for the manicurist and an ottoman for the client's feet as well as water basins, towels, toenail clippers, astringents, and antiseptics.

RETAIL SERVICES

Retail services involve the sale of products such as cleansers, toners, astringents, makeup, and beauty care items to clients for their use at home (Figure 4-7). Sales of these items can add significantly to your

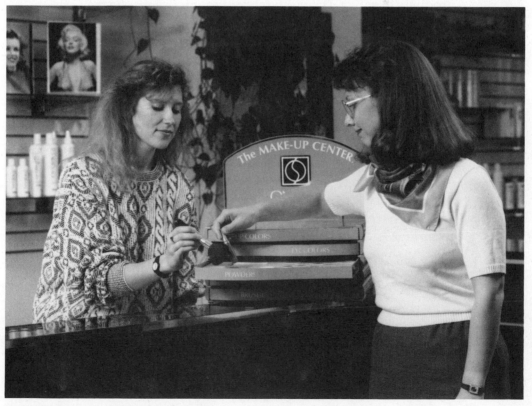

FIGURE 4-7 Retail sales

profitability. In addition, they can help reinforce the perception of quality of the other services you offer. They are the "finishing touch," so to speak. Sales are made to both men and women. (Retail operations are discussed in Chapter 13.)

Retail sales require little capital equipment, but you must stock sufficient inventory to meet your customers' needs. The items can be sold by an unlicensed individual and may offer a way to keep your receptionist or other designated salesperson busy. Little formal training is required, but the salesperson should be able to discuss the characteristics and use of the products, and training or experience in retail selling is helpful.

EQUIPMENT   Capital equipment includes shelves, display cases, and a cash register. Noncapital equipment includes ledgers to record sales and keep track of inventory. Supplies include adequate stocks of products to sell and sales literature about those products.

MISCELLANEOUS

In addition to the equipment you need for the services you offer in your salon, there is a body of equipment that you may need no matter what form your salon takes. These include a desk and chair for the receptionist, reception room chairs and tables, umbrella stands, coat racks, signage, ashtrays, wastebaskets and trash containers, brooms, mops and buckets, light fixtures, heaters and air conditioners, tables and chairs for staff lunch and breaks, rest room fixtures, storage bins, and office equipment such as filing cabinets, desks and chairs, and a computer and printer.

As this chapter shows, you can offer a tremendous variety of services in your skin and body care salon. As indicated, each requires specific equipment, although the list here is illustrative and not meant to be comprehensive. And each service has its own licensing and training requirements, as well. Complete information on specific requirements is available from your state board of cosmetology.

You can shape your salon as your abilities, interests, and pocketbook allow. But you have to consider your choices carefully, always keeping an eye to their profitability with your clientele in your area of operation.

SUMMARY

Your profitability will depend on the range of services you offer in your salon. The services you choose to offer depend on a number of factors: your interests and abilities, the clientele you expect to serve, and the demographics of the area in which your salon is located.

In your skin care salon, the services you offer may be categorized as skin and body care services, hair removal services, makeup application and cosmetics services, and nail services. In addition, you may sell products for home use at retail. Each type of service you offer has its own special requirements for training, licensing, and equipment.

SKIN CARE SALON DESIGN

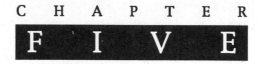

C H A P T E R
F I V E

The environment in which you provide your various skin and body care services is just as important as the quality of the services themselves. In many ways, your salon design, the environment you create, will shape the quality of your services. The facilities in your salon, its size, layout, and organization all contribute to the ease with which you, your estheticians, and other employees will be able to work and will raise the comfort level of the clients. An effective, attractive, pleasing design will go a long way toward instilling confidence in your customers.

A skin and body care salon, perhaps more than any other service business, relies on a bond of trust forged between client and esthetician. Your salon design creates the atmosphere that helps forge this bond. When your client enters a bright, clean, cheerful place and is greeted with warmth and friendship, he or she will be confident about receiving the best services and will reward you with repeat business.

The environment inside and outside of your salon says a lot about you and your operation. Effective beauty and health care is as much a psychological function as it is a physical one. The better the surroundings, the happier the client will be with the quality of the care he or she receives. A quality environment will help attract clients and, just as importantly, help keep those clients. And no salon, no matter how accomplished the staff, can function without customers.

THE PHYSICAL ENVIRONMENT

Location

Good salon design starts with the site, so consider your location carefully. It is important to choose the right neighborhood for the salon. The neighborhood demographics, that is, the characteristics of the people who live and work in the neighborhood, should match the characteristics of the clientele you are trying to reach. The people in the area of the salon should have the inclination to utilize the services of a skin and body care salon, and they should have the means to purchase the services at the prices you charge.

You should also make sure the site is zoned for commercial use and that there are no undue restrictions that may limit how you conduct your business. Find out if there are any changes planned for the area, such as new construction or rerouting of traffic patterns, by checking with your local zoning commission and with the local merchants' association, if there is one.

The salon should be readily accessible and easily reached by both automobile and public transportation. Location in a shopping center, mall, or along a major highway usually meets these criteria. As it is important to have accessibility for the handicapped, first floor locations without steps are best.

Adequate parking facilities are vital. Space available for parking should be ample and well lighted at night. It should be an easy and safe walk from the parking area or from public transportation stops into the salon. The salon, as well, should be well lighted at night, both for patron safety and for high visibility from the street. If you have to, consider leasing extra outdoor space to use for parking. The importance of parking facilities cannot be overstated.

Signage

Signage is also important, both for people who are looking for the salon and for attracting passers-by. Your signs are your first line of communication with your customers. They direct customers to your salon, give them essential information about your salon, and project and build an image for your salon.

The signs should indicate the services available, either reflected in the name of the salon or contained in a phrase after it. For best visibility, outside signs should be internally illuminated with large letters for easy readability. The sign's design should be tasteful, not garish, to reflect the professionalism of the salon. It should make the salon look like a salon, not like a used-car lot. Make sure you check the sign ordinances in your community and be aware of any restrictions on signage in your lease.

Window signs should be either neon or well lighted, so they'll be readily visible both day and night. Like the external signs, they should be tastefully designed and arranged in the window to avoid a cluttered appearance. They should allow free vision into the salon from the outside, as activity inside the salon can also be a drawing point for passers-by.

Your signs are a major investment, but, properly designed and constructed, they will last for a long time. Don't cut corners with your signage. Consult with a competent sign company and follow their recommendations. Once your signs are installed, maintain them properly. Keep them clean and replace burned out bulbs or damaged parts promptly. A worn out, unkempt sign indicates to customers that you don't care enough about your business to provide first-rate services.

Hire a good graphic designer to design your sign and your logo. Many small sign companies don't have designers on staff and lack the capability to develop good designs. Remember the importance of image. It is money well spent to have a good design for your sign to protect and enhance the image of your salon.

Interior Design

The interior design of the salon depends largely on the range of skin and body care services you offer. The internal facilities must be well thought out and designed to give you the maximum flexibility and efficiency.

The decor you choose should reflect the image you're trying to create. Your choices are virtually unlimited. But make sure to create an attractive, inviting ambience. Keep the color schemes harmonious. Keep the furniture and fixtures in good condition. And make sure the salon is always spotlessly clean. You might consider hiring a competent interior decorator to help with the design. Make sure, however, that he or she has experience in designing salons.

COLOR IN SALON DESIGN   Color is an important aspect of your salon design. The efficient use of color will give your salon its unique ambience. In addition to their decorative function, the colors you choose will have a definite psychological effect on your staff and your clients so pick your color scheme carefully.

Different light sources have different color casts, depending on the color temperature of the source. Incandescent lamps, for example, tend toward the red end of the spectrum; fluorescent lights tend toward the blue end. Even daylight changes color. Depending on the time of day and weather conditions, it can vary from red to blue.

Colors also have temperature. They can be thought of in terms of warm, neutral, or cool. Colors containing a predominance of red or yellow tend to be warm; those containing a predominance of blue or green tend to be cool. White, gray, and black are neutral.

The aspects of color—hue, value, intensity, and temperature—are important considerations when choosing the colors to use in your salon decor. While colors can be combined in almost limitless numbers, not all combinations are pleasing. Some combinations are harmonious; others clash.

There is also a definite psychology of color, both in how they are perceived and in the moods they evoke. Color is as much a factor of human perception as it is a physical concept. People see colors differently. A shade of red, for example, will look different to a person with blue eyes than it does to a person with brown eyes. In addition, a given color is seen differently depending on the context in which it is viewed. Thus, a bright red dot on a lighter red field would appear more intense than it actually is. However, that same bright red dot on a darker red field would appear less intense than it actually is.

Light or bright colors appear to come forward, or advance. Dark or dull colors appear to move backward, or recede. This perception of color is sometimes used to create the illusion of more or less space. So you can utilize color to make your salon feel larger or more cozy. Likewise, some colors reflect their hue into adjacent areas, giving those areas overtones of that hue. In addition to color, judicious placement of mirrors will also make a small space seem larger. Remember, however, that mirrors will also reflect colors.

You can also adjust space with placement of lights and lighting fixtures. Spotlights can highlight areas of the salon and give them more prominence. Conversely, shading areas can reduce their prominence. Thus, with light, you can direct attention where and when you want. You can also create different effects by changing the color temperature of the lighting, for example, with warm light in the reception areas and daylight lighting in the work areas.

The psychological effect of color has long been known. Different colors are associated with different states of emotion. We are "blue" when we feel sad; we are "green" with envy; we refer to a coward as "yellow"; we "see red" with anger. The color used in the immediate environment can have subtle effects on mood and behavior. Green, for example, is soothing and tranquil and is appropriate for use in treatment rooms and reception areas. Blue promotes a feeling of spaciousness and can be used in smaller, more confined areas such as rest rooms. Yellow is cheerful and stimulating and can be used in consultation rooms and retail areas.

THE PSYCHOLOGICAL ENVIRONMENT

The psychological environment of the salon must also be well thought out. The ambiance, the "feel" of the salon, is just as vital to the success of the operation as the physical layout. Obviously, the salon must be well equipped and well maintained. It must also be comfortable and allow the client to relax.

The setting, no less than the demeanor of the staff, must radiate a feeling of professionalism and inspire confidence on the part of the client. A clean, modern, well-organized salon justifies the client's expectations that he or she will get full value for the dollars spent. And a client who leaves the salon satisfied will most likely be a source of repeat business and of referrals.

THE IDEAL SKIN CARE SALON

As with most aspects of skin and body care, there is no one best way to design a salon. Ideas must be modified to suit the situation and the particular needs of the individual owner. Very few situations will reach the ideal. The best that can be hoped for is to approach that ideal. The suggestions contained in this chapter are meant to stimulate creative thought about the needs of the salon and are not intended to be considered as absolutes. Obviously, you will design your salon to meet the constraints of your location, your building, and your pocketbook. Figure 5-1 shows one possible approach to salon layout.

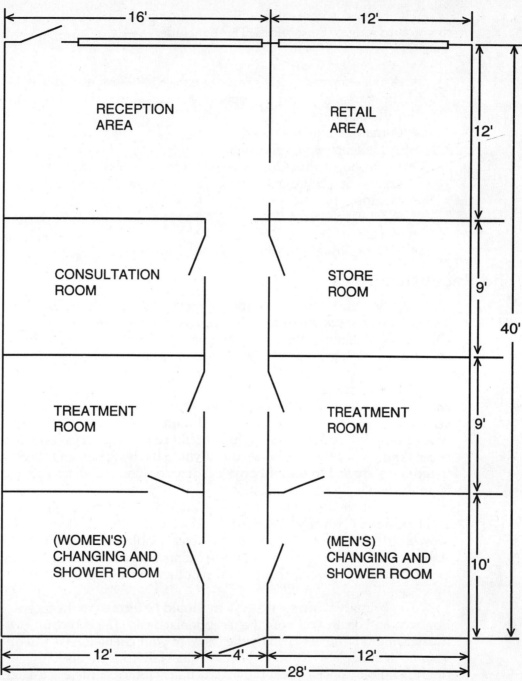

FIGURE 5-1 Salon layout

The ideal skin care salon will have a number of areas, each devoted to its specific services. These include:

- A reception area.
- A skin care area, consisting of a consultation room and one or more treatment rooms, especially if the salon will expand into full body care.
- A manicuring area.
- A makeup application area.
- Restroom facilities for men and women, with shower and changing facilities if full body care services are offered.
- A supply room.
- A retail sales area.
- An office.
- An employee lunchroom and break area.

The Reception Area

The reception area is one of the most important areas in the salon. It is the first area the client sees and sets the tone for his or her visit. It should be as roomy as the salon configuration allows, but should be spacious enough to hold six to ten people comfortably (Figure 5-2). Privacy is not a consideration in this part of the salon.

The floor should be carpeted and the walls should be papered in bright, cheerful colors. The room should be well lit with either fluorescent or incandescent lamps. Daylight illumination should be allowed when possible. Curtains or awnings should be provided, however, for those hours when the sun shines directly into the reception area, both to reduce glare and to prevent physical deterioration and discoloring from the sun's ultraviolet radiation.

Furnishings should include a desk and chair for the receptionist and a number of comfortable chairs for the clients. If they fit without crowding, one or more end tables and a coffee table may be added. Ashtrays should be provided for those clients who must smoke. Smoking should not be permitted in any other area of the salon, however.

The primary salon sound system should be located in the reception area and controlled from the receptionist desk. The choice of music should be determined by the tastes of your clientele, not you or your cosmetologists. If you like heavy metal but your clients like opera, you play opera. Generally, particularly if the clientele is mixed, middle-of-the-road or "easy listening" music will be most appropriate.

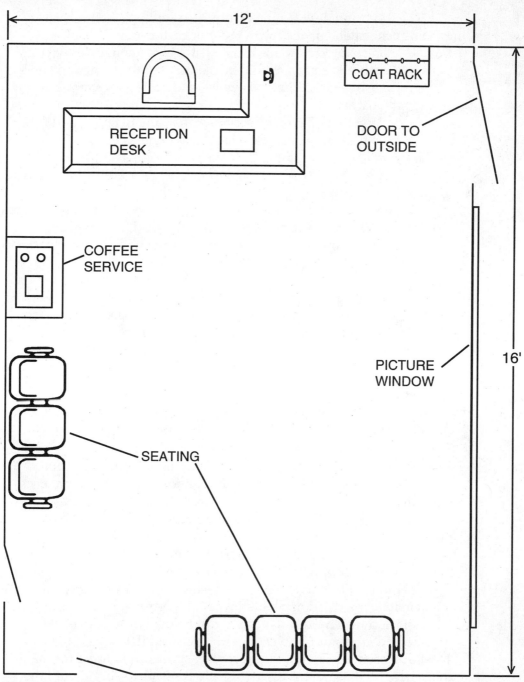

FIGURE 5-2   Reception area layout

The reception desk should be outfitted with a telephone, an appointment calendar, and a computer or cash register. A separate pay telephone should be made available for client convenience. Coat racks and umbrella stands should be placed near the front door, and rubber or plastic mats should be available to protect the carpet during inclement weather.

Complementary beverage service, consisting of coffee and selected herb teas, may be made available as long as the service area can be kept neat and sanitary. Only disposable cups and stirrers should be used. Sugar and artificial sweeteners should be available in single serving packets.

Current magazines of interest to both men and women should be provided for the clients' use. When not being read, the magazines should be kept in magazine racks. Product literature and articles on current fashions, skin and nail care should also be available in the reception area.

Display materials, product posters, and the like should be kept in the reception area. Unless there is a separate retail sales area elsewhere in the salon, retail sales should take place here also. (In this case, it will be necessary to add display counters and shelves.)

The Skin Care Area

THE CONSULTATION ROOM   The consultation room, which may also double as an office, is the area in which the client is first introduced to skin care (Figure 5-3). Pre-treatment and post-treatment discussions with the client take place here. Using a separate room for these discussions frees the treatment room for more productive use. Since the consultation room is also an area in which the client spends time, it must project the same aura of professionalism that the treatment room projects.

The minimum size for the consultation room should be nine feet by twelve feet, although it should be larger if a number of files are kept there. The floor may be covered with either carpeting or tile. Walls may be panelled or covered with a high-quality wallpaper. The decor should match that established for the salon as a whole.

The room should be well lit with overhead fluorescent lighting. The fluorescent tubes should deliver full-spectrum lighting for maximum benefit. It is not necessary to have controllable lighting in the consultation room, since it will not be necessary to dim the lights at

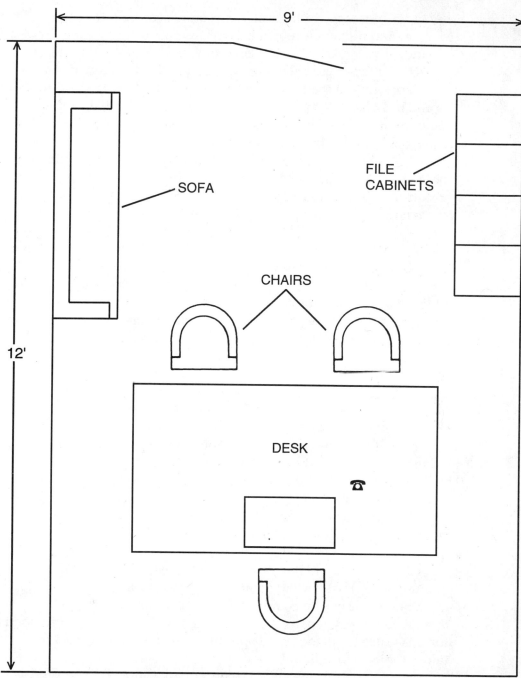

FIGURE 5-3   Consultation room layout

any time. Nor is there any need for a sound system in the room. The room should be soundproofed as much as possible, however, to mask outside noises. Like the treatment room, privacy is important to protect client confidentiality and to keep the client's mind at ease.

A desk and a chair for the esthetician will be needed, and there should be at least two padded chairs, one for the client, the other for a companion if the client chooses to bring one. One or more filing cabinets will be needed for record storage.

Diplomas and licenses should be displayed on the consultation room walls, along with charts and posters illustrating various aspects of skin care. A tastefully done, low-key product display is also appropriate here.

THE TREATMENT ROOM   The treatment room is the key to the skin care section's operation (Figure 5-4). This is where the work will actually be done and is the area that will leave the deepest impression on the client. It must be clean, well-appointed, quiet, and private.

Among the factors to be considered in the design of the treatment room are size and shape. The treatment room should be large enough for one client, the esthetician, and the equipment and supplies to fit comfortably. The optimum size is nine feet by twelve feet. Smaller than this will be cramped and uncomfortable; larger will leave too much empty space, which can also be uncomfortable. The room's shape should be rectangular.

As it is also important that the room allow privacy for the client, a door should screen the inside from view. A sign on the door should indicate when a treatment is in progress, to prevent anyone other than the esthetician from entering. If there are separate changing rooms, the client should be able to go directly from the changing room to the treatment room without passing through more public areas of the salon.

The room should be designed to allow ease of cleaning and maintenance. Fixtures and equipment should be able to be wiped clean and be disinfected, and electrical and water lines should be accessible for easy repair. A covered wastebasket should be provided for trash (use liners for easy disposal) in addition to a covered container for used towels and smocks.

The room's decor should be conservative, modern, and professional. Walls should be panelled or covered with high-quality

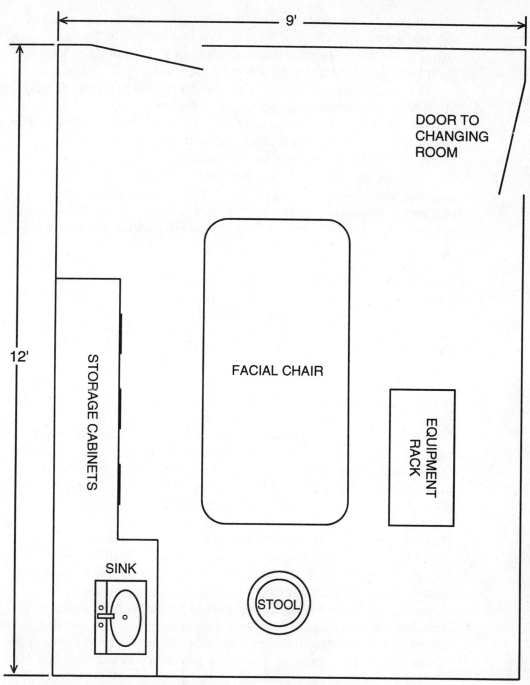

9'

DOOR TO
CHANGING
ROOM

12'

STORAGE CABINETS

FACIAL CHAIR

EQUIPMENT RACK

SINK

STOOL

FIGURE 5-4 Treatment room layout

wallpaper that should be washable. The ceiling should be acoustic tile, white or off-white. The floor should be tiled as tile floors are easier to clean and sanitize than carpeting or wood flooring. Wall and floor treatments should complement each other.

Decorations should be tasteful and contribute to the air of relaxation needed. Estheticians' licenses and diplomas should be displayed in the treatment room only if they are not shown in the consultation room. Product displays should be minimized as the treatment room is no place for the hard product sell.

Proper lighting is important to the treatment room. Overall lighting should be furnished by one or more ceiling-mounted or recessed fluorescent fixtures, shielded by diffusers. Bare bulbs should not be used. The fixtures should be placed to provide even illumination throughout the room.

These lights will be used before a treatment begins and after it is completed. During the treatment, however, the overhead lights will be off. At this point, there should be a source of indirect lighting, controlled by a dimmer switch to regulate the amount of light in the room. While a treatment is in progress, the overall light in the room should be subdued. It should be low enough to contribute to the feeling of relaxation, yet high enough to allow the esthetician to function. The only other light source needed in the treatment room is the magnifying lamp for analysis and manual extraction. While using the Wood's lamp, the room should be totally dark.

Enough electrical power should be available in the treatment room to handle all of the equipment used. There should be enough outlets in the room so that each appliance can be plugged into its own outlet without the need for extension cords. If possible, the power should be broken up into more than one circuit to prevent overloading. All outlets should be grounded to prevent electric shock, and circuit breakers should be easily accessible for quick resetting.

Hot and cold running water should be available in the room to allow mixing dry products, for washing implements, and for dampening towels. Heat and air conditioning should be adjustable. The room should be slightly on the warm side for the client's maximum comfort. Heating and cooling vents should have baffles to prevent air currents from blowing directly on the client or from interfering with jets of steam from the vaporizer. Adequate ventilation is important. It may be desirable to have an exhaust fan in the room to remove unwanted odors.

Equipment and supplies should be arranged to minimize excess motion on the part of the esthetician, which allows him or her to work in a more professional manner. The facial chair will be placed in the center of the room with unimpeded access to all four sides. The facial equipment should be placed around the chair so it can be put into use easily and efficiently. Supply cabinets should be closed to keep out dust and dirt. Supplies should be organized so the most used items will be within closest reach. Towels should be kept in a closed, dry area. Sufficient counter area for holding implements and products being used during the treatment should be available as well.

The room should be quiet and insulated from extraneous noise from other areas of the salon or the street. The treatment room should have its own sound system, both to help mask outside noise and to allow playing relaxing music. No telephone should be allowed in the treatment room.

The Manicuring Area

The manicure area may be open to general view from the public areas (Figure 5-5). You will need a space at least six feet by six feet. The advantage to such an area is its visibility. Clients waiting for skin care services will see manicures and pedicures being given and you may be able to sell additional services to them. Privacy for these services is not a factor, but the space shouldn't be crowded.

The area should be equipped with a manicure table, a chair for the client, and a chair or stool for the manicurist, along with an ottoman or low stool for pedicures. A free-standing cabinet for manicure supplies should be available in the area. Since there will be a lamp on the table, overhead lighting is not necessary. The ambient light level in the public areas should be sufficient, unless the corner is exceptionally dark.

If you have a separate room you can allocate for the nail services, you may utilize that but it should be well ventilated. Some nail services, for example acrylic nail applications, give off acrid fumes that may cause some discomfort. As with the rest of the salon, walls should be painted or papered and tastefully decorated; floors should be tiled for ease of cleaning. The room should be well lighted with fluorescent ceiling fixtures. The minimum room size should be eight feet by eight feet.

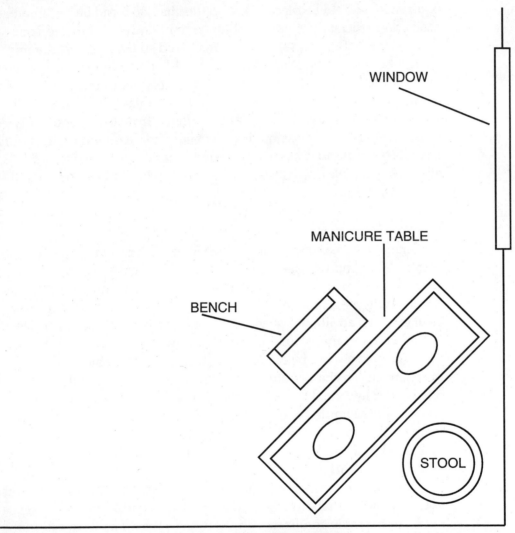

FIGURE 5-5   Manicure area layout

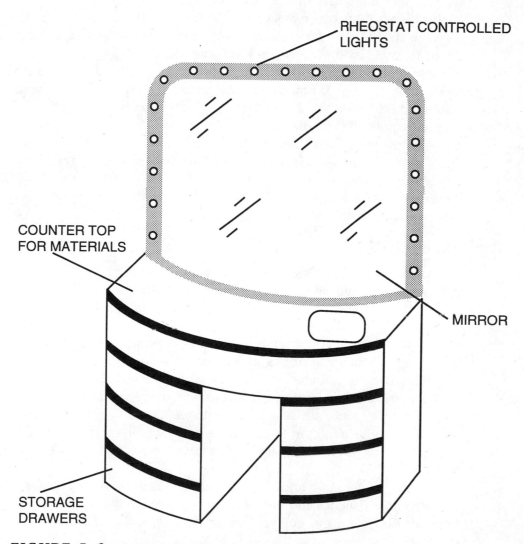

FIGURE 5-6   Makeup application area layout

The Makeup Application Area

The area you utilize for makeup application may be either a separate space in the public area or a separate room, possibly shared with another service, such as manicuring (Figure 5-6). The space should be between six and eight feet square. Walls should be a neutral color or white, to avoid casting color shadows onto the client's face while the makeup is being applied. Overhead lighting should be controlled by a rheostat so it can be dimmed or turned off during application, to avoid color contamination. While the area may be set off in a corner, it should be partially screened and be semiprivate.

The makeup artist's station should be ringed with incandescent lights that are controlled by a rheostat to simulate different lighting conditions, ranging from daylight to evening. The counter should have drawers for supplies. A hydraulic chair may be used at the makeup application station.

Restroom Facilities

The salon should have separate restroom facilities for men and women that should be large enough for clients to change from street clothes into treatment smocks (Figure 5-7). If facials and waxing are the only skin care services offered in the salon, shower facilities will not be necessary. If full-body treatments or massage are available, however, the shower facilities are a must.

The rooms should be divided into wet and dry areas. For cleaning and maintenance ease, wall surfaces in the wet areas should be ceramic tile. Floor surfaces in the wet areas should be nonslip tile for safety. Wall surfaces in the dry areas may be painted in bright restful colors or papered with water-resistant wallpaper, and floors may be tiled.

Only shower stalls and toilets should be placed in the wet areas of the rooms. Benches and mirrors may be placed in the dry areas. Lighted mirrors for makeup application should be placed in the ladies' changing room.

The rooms should be well lit with overhead fluorescent lighting, and fixtures in wet areas should be shielded from contact with water. Adequate supplies of hot water should be available. Adequate ventilation, especially in the wet areas, should be provided. Exhaust fans may be necessary.

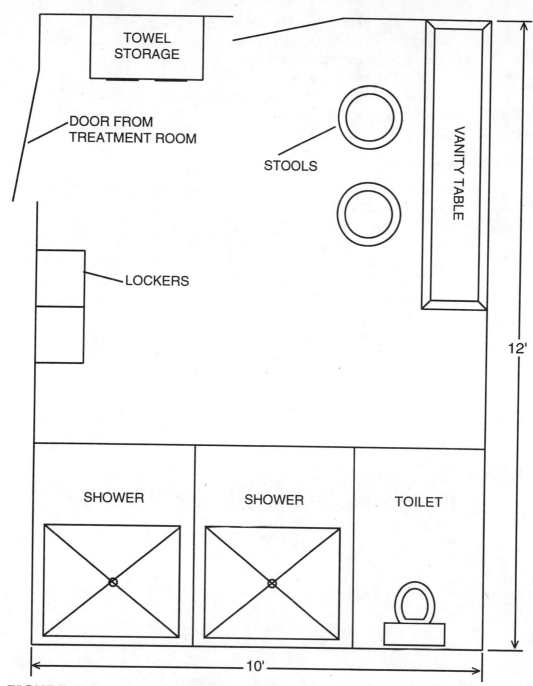

FIGURE 5-7   Restroom facilities layout

Secure lockers should be provided for clients' valuables. Towels and smocks should be stored in clean, dry cabinets, and covered containers for used smocks and towels should be provided.

Body cleansers and shampoos should be provided in the shower. (Preferably, these would be samples of products that are for sale in the salon.) Since the skin care section discourages the use of soap, it should not be provided in the shower room.

Supply Room

The supply room is the area where treatment and retail products are stored and from which they are drawn for use or sale (Figure 5-8). The room does not have to be large, but it must be well organized, with adequate shelving and cabinetry to store all of the salon's stocks of products and consumable materials. It should be well lit and have adequate ventilation. Decor is not important but the room should be kept clean. The door or storage cabinets should be lockable, and only employees should have access to the supply room.

There should also be an inventory control system. As products are received by the salon, they should be entered into a log. When products are taken from the supply room, they should be signed out. Stock should be rotated so the oldest products are used first.

Record keeping is important to the profitability of the salon. A good inventory control system lets the manager know which products sell well and which do not. It will also reduce waste and pilferage.

Retail Sales Area

The retail sales area is an important part of the salon (Figure 5-9). It is a good profit center, generating cash that can be reinvested in the salon. In addition, having products available at the retail level serves as an additional incentive for getting the client to follow the recommended home regimes for skin care. The easier it is for the client to get those recommended products, the more likely he or she is to use them.

The retail area should be roomy and visible from other areas of the salon and the outside. Floors may be carpeted, and walls should be bright and cheerful. The room should be well lit for maximum visibility. Spotlights may be strategically located to highlight specific products.

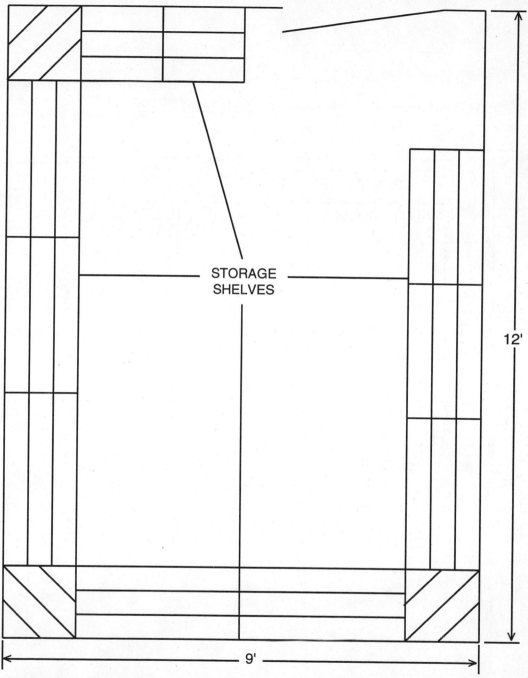

STORAGE
SHELVES

12'

9'

FIGURE 5-8   Supply room layout

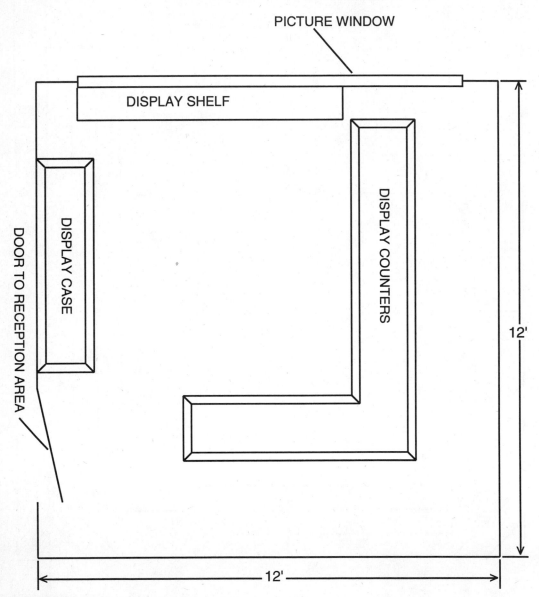

PICTURE WINDOW

DISPLAY SHELF

DISPLAY CASE

DISPLAY COUNTERS

DOOR TO RECEPTION AREA

12'

12'

FIGURE 5-9   Retail area layout

Display products in cases that allow easy visibility yet discourage shoplifting. Cases should be kept clean. Glass surfaces should be kept free of fingerprints.

Stock should be kept clean and periodically rearranged to present a new look to the area. All products should be clearly priced. Records should be kept of client purchases.

Office Area

A private office area is important to the salon. This is where you will keep records, can interview prospective employees, and will conduct the business aspects of the salon. It doesn't have to be very large, nor does it have to be furnished ostentatiously.

The minimum area should be approximately ten feet by ten feet and well lighted with fluorescent fixtures. Walls may be papered or painted and the floor may be carpeted or tiled. The room should be well ventilated. Furniture should include a desk and chair, one or two other chairs, and locking file cabinets for your records.

The desk should be equipped with a telephone and in-and-out boxes for correspondence. You may want to have a computer terminal in the office, too. Walls should be tastefully decorated with posters or other artwork.

The office door should have a lock and a sign identifying it as the office and prohibiting entry except by authorized personnel.

Employee Lunchroom and Break Area

It is important to provide a separate area where employees can go for breaks and for lunch. There are two reasons for this. One, it improves employee morale. They have a relatively quiet place to get away from the hustle and bustle of a busy salon. Two, it preserves the atmosphere of the salon for the customers. You do not want to have the employees lounging in the salon working areas when they're on their break or lunch period. Nor do you want them eating there, which is both unsanitary and unsightly.

Although not the most important area of the salon, it should be more than just an afterthought. It should be large enough for comfort, at least ten by fifteen feet or larger, depending on the size of your staff. The room should be bright, with windows, if possible, and well ventilated. The walls should be painted or papered with washable paper and the floors should be of tile for easy cleaning. There should be adequate fluorescent lighting and electrical outlets.

The break area should be furnished with a table and enough chairs for everyone. If the room is large enough for all of your employees, you might want to hold staff meetings and training sessions there. You might want to have a television set with a VCR so staff members can view training videotapes.

There should also be a sink with hot and cold running water for rinsing dishes, and closed cabinets to hold tableware and foodstuffs. You might install a microwave oven in the room for the convenience of the employees, but be careful of cooking food in the room. You don't want cooking odors to permeate the rest of the salon. If any cooking is done in the room, there should be an exhaust fan to remove odors.

In addition, you should have lockers where the employees can secure their personal belongings. Walls may be decorated with photographs or posters illustrating various skin care salon techniques. Many of these items are available from equipment and product manufacturers. You should also have a bulletin board to post notices and employee information.

If your state regulations allow, you may also install a washer and dryer in this room for laundering towels and smocks. Be aware, however, that some states do not allow salons to launder their own towels and other washable goods. Check with your state board of cosmetology to determine what rules apply.

SUMMARY

The environment created by your skin and body care salon can have a profound effect on the quality of the services you offer. A proper environment makes your customers more comfortable and more confident in your abilities.

Location is an important factor. The salon must be easily accessible with adequate parking. Handicapped access is also important. The interior decor and colors should reflect the image you are trying to create for the salon.

Rooms and work areas should be designed with a view to their efficient functioning and should be as spacious as necessary for the services that will be provided in them. As much as the physical facilities will permit, various service areas should be separated. Privacy is especially important in consultation and treatment rooms. The employees should have a private area where they can take breaks and have their meals.

THE SALON AND THE LAW

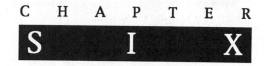

C H A P T E R
SIX

In the course of conducting your business, you'll find that your salon is subject to a myriad of laws and regulations, promulgated by agencies at the local, state, and federal levels. Some of these deal specifically with the cosmetology industry. Others deal with all businesses. Like it or not, these laws exist and must be obeyed. Failure to comply with the provisions of the various laws and ordinances can have severe consequences. You risk heavy fines, imprisonment, even the loss of your business. It is up to you to be aware of all of the laws and regulations that apply to your salon. Ignorance of the law is not an excuse.

It helps if you don't view the agencies that promulgate the regulations as adversaries, but consider them allies. These agencies exist to protect the public. In this function, they can provide substantial help to you by providing a legal framework in which you can conduct your business and by helping you conduct your business in a fair and equitable manner that protects you, your staff, and your customers.

FEDERAL AGENCIES

There are many government agencies that affect the cosmetology business, either directly or indirectly. On the federal level, the most important of this alphabet soup of rule-making agencies that concern

**CHECKLIST 6-1
FEDERAL AGENCIES**

1. **Food and Drug Administration (FDA)**—Responsible for monitoring the safety and effectiveness of cosmetics; enforces the standards of the Food, Drug and Cosmetic Act.
2. **Federal Trade Commission (FTC)**—Enforces laws that regulate competitive practices; sets rules for the sale of franchise operations; prevents manufacture and sale of counterfeit products.
3. **Internal Revenue Service (IRS)**—Raises revenue for the federal government; promulgates and enforces tax laws.
4. **Immigration and Naturalization Service (INS)**—Issues work permits for legal aliens and prevents illegal aliens from working.
5. **Small Business Administration (SBA)**—Responsible for helping small businesses.
6. **Environmental Protection Agency (EPA)**—Responsible for protecting the environment; establishes rules for handling hazardous waste materials.
7. **Occupational Safety and Health Administration (OSHA)**—Responsible for assuring safety in the workplace.
8. **Wage and Hour Division of the Department of Labor**—Enforces the provisions of the Fair Labor Standards Act.
9. **Equal Employment Opportunities Commission (EEOC)**—Responsible for enforcing antidiscrimination laws.

your salon are the Food and Drug Administration (FDA), the Federal Trade Commission (FTC), the Internal Revenue Service (IRS), the Immigration and Naturalization Service (INS), the Small Business Administration (SBA), the Environmental Protection Agency (EPA), the Occupational Safety and Health Administration (OSHA), the Wage and Hour Division of the Department of Labor, and the Equal Employment Opportunities Commission (EEOC).

The Food and Drug Administration

The FDA is a regulatory agency charged with making sure that a wide range of products, from medical devices, drugs, and food to cosmetics, meet the standards of the Food, Drug and Cosmetic Act and that these products are both safe and effective. The agency tests and approves products and has the authority to remove from the marketplace products that don't meet standards. It can also refer cases to the Justice Department for prosecution in cases of fraud.

Many ingredients used in foods, drugs, and cosmetics must go through a rigorous certification process before the FDA will allow their use. Colorants, which give a product its characteristic color, fall into this category. Vegetable, mineral, or animal dyes or pigments may be used without specific government approval. These compounds and chemicals usually fall under an FDA classification known as GRAS, Generally Recognized As Safe. Coal tar derivative dyes, however, must undergo a long and expensive certification process before they can go into skin care products. Certified colorants are listed as FD&C (Food, Drug and Cosmetic) colors, D&C colors, or ext. D&C colors. FD&C colors can be used in food, drugs, and cosmetics. D&C colors may only be used in drugs and cosmetics. Ext. D&C colors are for external use only in drugs and cosmetics.

The agency has the responsibility to challenge claims made for products under its jurisdiction and to require substantiation for those claims. For example, the FDA is actively disputing the assertions some manufacturers of skin care products are making about the anti-aging capabilities of their products. If these manufacturers cannot prove their claims to the FDA's satisfaction, they will be forced to withdraw the products. If they do not withdraw the products voluntarily, the FDA has the authority to seize the products and bring the manufacturers into court.

By law, the Food and Drug Administration also has jurisdiction over packaging and labeling. Packaging cannot contain unsubstantiated claims about the product's effectiveness. Any information contained on the package must be factual. In addition, cosmetic products must list all ingredients on the label. The ingredients are listed in descending order according to the amount of the ingredient contained in the product. It is not necessary, however, to list the actual amount of each substance. Because of the proprietary nature of fragrances, specific components of the fragrance do not have to be listed.

The FDA also provides materials for consumer education, designed to keep consumers aware of the safety and efficacy of the products they purchase. The agency's monthly magazine, *The FDA*

Consumer, available by subscription from the FDA, is an excellent source of consumer information. In addition, the agency distributes a wide range of consumer oriented pamphlets through the government bookstores.

The Federal Trade Commission

The FTC regulates commerce in the United States and is responsible for enforcing laws that prevent unfair competitive practices. The agency helps maintain a level playing field so businesses can compete fairly. The FTC has little direct influence on the cosmetology business.

There are two areas where you may have dealings with the FTC, however. The first involves franchises. The agency sets rules for the sale of franchise operations. All franchise operators must abide by a set of comprehensive reporting regulations when they promote and sell the franchises. These laws were enacted to protect franchise purchasers. If you are thinking about buying a salon franchise, check with the FTC for a copy of the laws.

The FTC is also responsible for preventing the manufacture and distribution of counterfeit products. This is a major problem in the salon industry. Many well-known national brands of cosmetic products have been counterfeited. While these fakes are less expensive than the legitimate item, in many cases they are of inferior quality and may be unsafe to use. Also, it is illegal to knowingly purchase counterfeit products and sell them in your salon as the real thing. If you suspect a supplier is trying to sell you counterfeit products, contact the FTC.

The Internal Revenue Service

The IRS is the principal agency responsible for raising revenues for the federal government. It enforces federal tax codes and collects the taxes through a complex and constantly changing set of rules. You must be concerned with a number of taxes, such as income taxes on profits, withholding of employee's taxes, Social Security taxes, and self-employment taxes. There are very strict reporting requirements for the various kinds of taxes and severe penalties, which apply whether you make a mistake or deliberately evade payment, for failure to comply with the tax statutes. These taxes are described in IRS Publication 583, *Taxpayers Starting a Business.*

The complexity of the laws makes professional assistance necessary. Although it is not required by law, if you are in business, you should have an accountant handle this aspect for you. (Most of the applicable taxes are discussed in other chapters in this book.) In addition, the IRS offers a wide variety of booklets that explain the various provisions of the tax laws. Get copies and read them. You don't have to become an expert—that's why you have an accountant—but you should be aware of the various provisions of the laws. Make sure your accountant explains the tax laws that apply to your business.

The Immigration and Naturalization Service

Among its many responsibilities, the INS issues work permits to legal aliens and prevents illegal aliens from finding employment in this country. When you hire a new employee, you must comply with the provisions of the Immigration Reform and Control Act, which was passed in 1986. Under the provisions of this act, you may only hire U. S. citizens or legal aliens who are authorized to work in the United States. There are severe penalties, including fines and imprisonment, for violating this law.

You must have each employee fill out INS Form I-9, which verifies the employee's status, and you are responsible for the accuracy of the information on the form. That means you must check the documentation provided by the employee. The documentation may be in the form of a birth certificate, naturalization papers, or a green card issued by the INS. If you have any questions about the law, contact your local INS office.

The Small Business Administration

The SBA is responsible for helping small businesses, which are defined by their level of sales. For most service businesses, such as skin and body care salons, that level is set at annual sales of less than $2,000,000. The SBA is not a regulatory agency in the sense of the other agencies discussed here, but functions more to counsel small business owners and to provide assistance in finding capitalization, than in promulgating laws and regulations. Your local office of the SBA is an excellent source of information on management techniques. The agency publishes and distributes a wide variety of books and pamphlets of value to small business owners. Many of the functions of the SBA are covered in other chapters in this book.

The Environmental Protection Agency

As its name implies, the EPA is responsible for protecting the environment. One of the EPA's major concerns is the emission of volatile organic compounds (VOCs), which are the vapors released into the atmosphere when products made with petroleum-based solvents are used. At present the agency is mostly concerned with VOC control in manufacturing industries, but be aware that some of the products you use in your salon emit VOCs as well. These include nail polishes and nail polish removers, among others. If the agency decides to issue rules regulating the use of such salon products in the future, you will have to be aware of and follow them.

This agency also establishes rules for handling and disposing of hazardous waste materials. Many of the materials you handle in the salon can be considered hazardous, including a variety of solvents, disinfectants, and sanitary chemicals. Your concern with the EPA will be in how you dispose of these. How you handle them safely in the salon is a concern of OSHA.

Most of the waste products you generate in the salon will not be considered as hazardous, but some, such as alcohol and acetone, are classed as hazardous wastes. Be careful how you dispose of these. Do not pour them down the sink where they can enter the sewer system and contaminate the water supply. Similarly, items commonly used in skin care services, such as used lancets, cotton, and gauze, that have been in contact with a client's blood or other body fluids may be considered as hazardous and should be disposed of according to EPA guidelines. Check with your local EPA office to see which of the agency's provisions apply to your salon, then follow those provisions.

Proper waste disposal procedures are important whether or not the waste is considered hazardous. During the course of a day's operations, the salon generates a considerable amount of waste, both recyclable and disposable. These must be handled safely and efficiently to avoid risk of contamination. Trash should not be allowed to accumulate in the salon, but should be periodically bagged in heavy duty plastic trash bags, tightly sealed, and disposed of according to local ordinances, either through municipal or private trash collection services or in legal landfills.

The Occupational Safety and Health Administration

OSHA, responsible for assuring safety in the workplace, has jurisdiction over manufacturing and nonmanufacturing businesses of all sizes, including salons. The agency has the authority to conduct surprise inspections at any business location and to levy fines for noncompliance with safety regulations.

Salons are now covered under OSHA and are required by law to maintain a safe working environment for their employees. Part of the law requires salons to develop a written Hazard Communication Standard to make sure employees are aware of hazardous materials they may be required to use. This standard includes a written hazard communication program that outlines the salon's hazard communications efforts and must be both available and understandable to all employees. The program must include a list of every hazardous chemical in use in the salon. This includes such chemicals as acetone, alcohol, and other solvents.

The salon must have on file Material Safety Data Sheets (MSDS), available from the manufacturers of the products, for all hazardous chemicals on site. In addition, any product that contains a hazardous chemical must so state on its label. The salon should maintain a roster of all products used, with complete ingredient information. In addition, the salon must establish an ongoing training program to teach employees the proper use and potential dangers of any products they utilize.

In addition to OSHA requirements, many states have enacted right-to-know laws, which mandate that employers must inform employees about hazardous materials in the workplace. These regulations must be followed, as well.

The Wage and Hour Division of the Department of Labor

The Wage and Hour Division of the Department of Labor enforces the provisions of the Fair Labor Standards Act, which sets minimum wages and overtime pay requirements and establishes standards for using child labor. As an employer, you must be aware of the provisions of this law, some of which may be applicable to your salon. Check with the office in your area. (The major provisions of the wage and hour laws are discussed in Chapter 10.)

The Equal Employment Opportunity Commission

The EEOC is responsible for enforcing antidiscrimination laws, especially as they apply to fair employment practices. These laws prohibit you, as an employer, from discriminating against any employee because of race, national origin, religion, age, sex, or sexual preference. They cover virtually all aspects of employment, from recruiting, hiring, compensation, and training to termination. Essentially, they mean you must treat all employees according to the same rules and standards. Discrimination in any form, whether intentional or unintentional, is illegal.

The major law in this area is Title VII of the Civil Rights Act of 1964, which addresses racial discrimination, though the law's jurisdiction is not limited to those matters. The law also addresses sex discrimination. You may not refuse to hire someone because of race or color. Likewise, you may not refuse to hire someone because of sex or sexual preference, unless sex is a bona fide concern of the position. For example, you can't turn down a male applicant for an esthetician's job, which can be done by either sex. You may, however, refuse employment to a male for a job performing bikini waxing. You also must pay the same to males and females who are doing the same job. This does not mean that you have to pay a new or inexperienced worker at the same rate as a more experienced worker with more seniority.

The Pregnancy Discrimination Act of 1978 supplements Title VII. According to this statute, you must give a pregnant employee the same rights and benefits as you give any other disabled employee.

Sexual harassment is also an important issue. You have the responsibility to make sure none of your employees is sexually harrassed by any other employee. Sexual harassment can be almost any form of unwelcome behavior ranging from off-color language or jokes to physical contact. If an employee claims he or she has been harassed, you must correct the situation. If you do not take the claim seriously, you can be held liable in court.

As with race, you can't refuse to hire people because of their country of origin, as long as they can legally work in this country. This provision of the law can be tricky, however, since according to the INS, you can't hire someone who is an illegal alien. It means you can't make the decision based on their appearance or because they have foreign accents.

Discrimination because of age is also illegal. The Age Discrimination in Employment Act of 1967 protects employees over forty years of age. You may not refuse to hire nor may you terminate an employee on the basis of age, unless age is a bona fide criterion for the job, such as a requirement for hard physical labor. There are no jobs in a beauty salon where age is relevant.

You may not discriminate against employees because of their religious beliefs or practices. By law, you must let them observe their religious traditions, unless those observances cause a hardship to your business or to other employees. Thus, for example, you must allow an employee who celebrates the Sabbath on Friday to have that day off, as long as the absence doesn't cause the salon any difficulty. But, be sure you can document that difficulty.

The various provisions of these antidiscrimination statutes are complicated. Nevertheless, failure to comply with them can have severe consequences. Make sure you understand your obligations under the law. Discuss the matter with your attorney. Contact your local EEOC field office for more complete information.

All of the agencies discussed here maintain field offices in major cities around the country. Anytime you have a question about how their rules and regulations apply to you, call and ask. Don't assume that you are or are not covered. Find out before you get into trouble. Agency rules vary widely, so it is best to ask and be guided by the information you are given by your attorney and by the agency.

STATE AGENCIES

Each state has a large number of agencies, which exist either to regulate business or to generate revenue from business. Some do both. Many of these agencies parallel the federal agencies and perform many of the same functions, but have jurisdiction only within the borders of the state. Sometimes the state laws conflict with or vary from federal laws. In these cases, as a general rule, you will be bound by the more strict of the statutes. The federal law does not necessarily supersede the state law.

As with the federal agencies, some of the state governing bodies affect salons directly; others are of only indirect concern. The agencies that you will mostly deal with are state boards of cosmetology, state

> ## CHECKLIST 6-2
> ## STATE AGENCIES
>
> 1. **State boards of cosmetology**—Responsible for regulating and licensing salons and cosmetologists.
> 2. **State department of labor**—Promulgates and enforces state labor laws and enforces workers' compensation and unemployment insurance laws.
> 3. **State department of revenue**—Responsible for raising revenues for the state; levies and collects taxes.

departments of labor, and state departments of revenue. In addition, you should be aware of state Consumer Protection Laws, usually enforced by the state's Attorney General's office.

Laws vary widely from state to state. Some states regulate businesses heavily; others virtually not at all. Enforcement of laws also varies from one state to another. Because of this, it is impossible to give a comprehensive description of state laws governing small business. As with the federal laws, penalties for breaking the laws can be severe, whether you break them intentionally or unintentionally. So make sure you know the laws that apply to you. To find out about the laws that cover your salon, consult with your attorney and contact the regulatory agencies within your state.

State Boards of Cosmetology

State boards of cosmetology are the primary regulatory and licensing agencies for salons as well as for cosmetologists. They make and enforce the rules for the cosmetology profession and establish standards for training and licensing technicians and for the licensing and conduct of salon businesses. They set the basic rules under which you may operate your salon.

For most jobs in your salon, employees will have to possess a valid license from the state board, which they will earn by completing an approved course with a specified number of hours and by taking a stringent written and practical examination. In addition, you must have a valid salon license to open your doors for business. In most states, an agent from the state board will inspect your salon before you are granted the license, and will periodically inspect the salon after that.

State board regulations vary from state to state. Be sure you are familiar with and understand all of the regulations of the board of cosmetology in your state.

State Department of Labor

Like its federal counterpart, the state department of labor is responsible for safeguarding the rights of the employees and for promulgating and enforcing labor laws. Thus, your state may have its own antidiscrimination statutes that supplement or expand upon the federal laws. Your state may also have its own OSHA statutes.

State labor departments also enforce workers' compensation and unemployment insurance laws. These are state, not federal, functions. Every state has laws covering workers' compensation, although the provisions vary from one state to another. In general, all states let employees who are injured on the job recover medical expenses and disability pay, regardless of who is at fault. The injury must have occurred during work, however. The laws do not allow the injured employee to sue the employer for negligence.

The various state laws determine which employees are covered and which are not and whether your salon is covered by the statutes. If your business is covered, you must carry workers' compensation insurance. Your state department of labor or your insurance agent will give you the information you need.

The state department of labor also administrates the unemployment compensation laws. Unemployment compensation pays benefits to employees who lose their jobs without good cause. So, for example, if you fire an employee because of lack of work, he or she may be eligible for compensation. If the employee quits or is fired for misconduct, he or she will not be eligible for those payments.

The amount of the benefit payments and the length of time the employee may collect vary from state to state. The funds come from taxes on employers.

State Department of Revenue

The state department of revenue is responsible for levying and collecting taxes, which finance state programs. Currently, only seven states do not tax business income. If your salon is in Alaska, Florida, Nevada, South Dakota, Texas, Washington, or Wyoming, and your business is organized as a sole proprietorship or a partnership, you

will not pay state tax on your business income. If you are incorporated, you can subtract Alaska, Florida, and South Dakota from the
list. All other states collect taxes on business earnings.

All states, including these seven, levy a host of other taxes on
businesses. So, regardless of your location, you may pay sales and use
taxes, property taxes, capital gains taxes, or others. Your accountant
will tell you which taxes apply in your state.

Sales and use taxes are levies against goods and services you sell.
Most states have sales and use taxes, but the rate and the goods and
services subject to the tax vary from state to state. Check with your
state department of revenue to learn the regulations in your area.

You must collect these taxes from the customers and forward the
money to the state. In essence, you are the state government's tax col-
lector. In some states, you will be allowed to deduct a small commission from the payments you collect as recompense. You must first get
a state sales tax number, which is your authorization to collect the
taxes. When you purchase taxable goods or services, your supplier
will charge you sales tax unless you have this number, which exempts
you from paying the sales tax. However, you must pay a use tax
instead. The use tax is based on the fair value of the goods and services you received. The difference is that you pay the tax directly to
the state agency instead of paying it through the supplier.

LOCAL AGENCIES

In addition to those of the federal and state agencies, you will also be
bound by the regulations and laws of a variety of local agencies.
Exactly what these will be depend, in part, on the type of municipality
in which your salon is located and on how your state regulates what
laws municipalities can pass. Generally, the larger the municipality,
the more laws and regulations you will face, and the more stringent
those laws will be.

First, you should know the kind of community in which you're
doing business. This sounds simple, but can be more complicated
than it seems. Each type of municipality is rather loosely defined. The
definitions are made more complicated by the fact that the denotations
change from one region of the country to another. So, for example,
what is referred to as a borough in one state, may be called a village in
another.

CHECKLIST 6-3
LOCAL AGENCIES

1. **License and inspection agencies**—Grant business licenses and permits; inspect businesses to make sure they meet local standards and building codes.
2. **Zoning commissions**—Regulate the types of businesses and their operation in local areas.
3. **Tax authorities**—Responsible for raising revenues for local communities; levy and collect taxes.

In general terms, the various forms of municipalities include counties, cities, towns, villages, boroughs, and hamlets. Except for counties, all these types of municipalities are incorporated; that is, they form a legal body with a legitimate government. A county is the largest territorial division of a state with a separate local government. Each county has a seat, usually a town within its borders, that is home to the government offices and county courthouse and is the base of the county's elected and appointed officials. A county will contain one or more incorporated municipalities and may contain rural or unincorporated areas, as well. In addition to their own laws and regulations, incorporated municipalities are subject to those of the county. Rural or unincorporated areas do not have their own governments, and are subject to the laws of the county.

A city is a municipality governed under a charter granted by the state. It is usually larger and more densely populated than a town or village. Some cities and counties are contiguous; that is, they occupy the same boundaries. For example, the city of Philadelphia and Philadelphia County cover the same geographical area. Most cities, however, are located within a county. A suburb is a small community or area located next to a city, but not covered by its charter or subject to its municipal laws. The suburb may be an incorporated municipality or unincorporated.

A town is an organized community that is usually smaller than a city but larger than a village. A village is an incorporated community that is larger than a hamlet. Either may be called a borough. A township is a larger unit that may contain one or more villages or hamlets.

Each municipality has agencies that exist to regulate business or to levy taxes. In the course of establishing or managing your salon, you will deal with a number of them, including license and inspection agencies, zoning commissions, and various tax authorities. The larger the municipality, the more of them will be involved with your business.

License and Inspection Agencies

In most municipalities, you will need to obtain a business license before you can open your salon. This is separate and different from the salon license granted by the state board of cosmetology. The business license is granted annually on payment of the licensing fees. License and inspection agencies also grant various permits, one-time licenses, that you will need if you want to make changes in or additions to your structure. The agencies also maintain staffs of inspectors, who will periodically visit and examine your business to make sure it meets the local standards and building codes.

Zoning Commissions

Most municipalities have zoning ordinances that regulate what kind of businesses may operate within its borders and where they may operate. The ordinances may also regulate the size and placement of signs, as well as other aspects of the physical facilities of the business. The ordinances are enforced by a zoning commission or board.

Zoning ordinances are important, and you must know which apply to you. If you violate them, you face fines or loss of the business. Make sure the location you choose to establish your salon is zoned for commercial use. Also, know what restrictions apply to building sizes, signs, lighting, parking, and any other details of your business. Find out before you invest in the location. Zoning commissions hold regularly scheduled meetings. Attend them and ask specific questions about the ordinances that apply to you.

Tax Authorities

In addition to the taxes you must pay to the federal government and to the state, you also face local taxes, levied by a number of tax authorities. These taxes may include business taxes on profits, school taxes levied by the school board, occupational taxes, head taxes, and wage taxes. You may even be responsible for taxes levied by communities other than the one in which your place of business is located. For example, if you live in one community and have your business in another, you may have to pay taxes to both. Like federal and state tax laws, local tax laws can be complicated. Make sure your accountant explains which apply to you.

Because of the great differences in laws from state to state and municipality to municipality, it is impossible to cover each adequately in one book. Rely on the advice of your attorney and accountant to make sure you comply with the regulations that are applicable to you and your salon.

SUMMARY

Like it or not, you will be subject to a host of laws and regulations, promulgated by a seemingly endless number of agencies on the federal, state, and local levels, when you operate your salon. Some of the agencies regulate all business; others are concerned only with cosmetology businesses and practices.

You must be aware of which agencies have an effect on your business and what laws and regulations apply to you. Failure to abide by the laws, whether you break the rules knowingly or inadvertently, can result in severe penalties.

You must be concerned with the tax laws promulgated by the IRS. Because of the complexity of the tax laws, it is a necessity to have an accountant handle these matters. Rely on him or her for advice in this area.

Some government agencies, such as the Small Business Administration, are chartered to help small businesses by providing advice and counsel and, in some cases, helping arrange for capital financing.

Many state agencies duplicate the functions of federal agencies. Where state regulations conflict with federal regulations, the more stringent statutes apply. State laws vary widely from one state to another, so make sure you are aware of which laws apply in the state in which you operate. You will probably be most affected by your local state board of cosmetology, which makes and enforces the rules for your profession. In addition, the community in which you operate may have its own licensing and taxing authorities.

LEGAL REQUIREMENTS

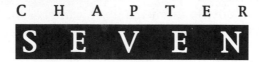

C H A P T E R
SEVEN

In the preceding chapter, the various laws and government bodies that affect the establishment and operation of your salon were discussed. That information provides you with a theoretical background. However, the laws set up by these various institutions have practical application to your business. To open and maintain your skin and body care salon, you must be aware of and follow these laws and procedures.

Starting and running your business encompasses far more than just getting your equipment, hanging out your sign, and opening your doors. You must first become a legal entity, registered to do business in your state and locality. You must get all of the permits and licenses required, and make sure you comply with all codes and ordinances that apply to your business. You must also make sure you are operating in compliance with the various laws that apply to all businesses. To further complicate matters, you must accomplish most of these tasks before you open for business.

FINDING LEGAL REPRESENTATION

Early in the planning stage, hire a competent attorney to help you through the legal hurdles. Just as you need the services of a qualified

CHECKLIST 7-1
CHOOSING AN ATTORNEY

When looking for an attorney:

1. Get recommendations.
2. Interview all prospective attorneys.
3. Look for experience in handling small businesses.
4. Check qualifications and experience.
5. Discuss your needs and expectations.
6. Check references.
7. Discuss fees and how they will be paid.

accountant and an obliging banker, so in this legalistic day and age, you need a good lawyer. Find an attorney the same way you find other advisors. Ask other business people for recommendations. Get recommendations from your local bar association. Ask your accountant and banker for suggestions.

A word of caution here. Many people view lawyers with an awe they don't have for other professional people, like accountants and bankers. Don't hold this attitude. There is no special mystique about the legal profession. A lawyer is a business person, just like you. Use the same judgmental criteria with the attorney that you use with anyone else.

Look for an attorney who has experience handling small business affairs. From your list of recommendations, choose a number who seem to fit your needs, then talk to them. Don't be afraid to ask for their qualifications and experience. Let them know what your needs and expectations are, and ask questions. Remember, in effect you are interviewing them with the idea of having them represent you. Be just as thorough in these interviews as you would be if you were interviewing candidates for a job in your salon. If the attorney objects to answering your questions, he or she is not the right lawyer for you.

You should probably look for a small local law firm. Attorneys in smaller firms will usually have more time to devote to your needs, and they will usually be less expensive. Large firms, on the other hand, devote most of their efforts to big businesses and, if they handle your affairs at all, will give the assignment to one of their junior people. You want to choose a law firm that will give you the care and consideration you deserve and are paying for, not one where you'll get buried under their "more important" clients. Remember the concept of customer service. You are that firm's customer and you deserve the same level of service that your clients expect and deserve from you.

Make sure the lawyer is familiar with the needs of small businesses and with laws and ordinances that affect business. Get references and check on them. After all, you will do this in choosing your accountant and banker. Why not for your lawyer, too? Also discuss fees. How will you pay your attorney? Will you pay an hourly rate or a flat rate? Can you ask for information over the telephone? If so, is a phone call charged at the same rate as an office visit? Know all of these things up front.

There are three ways to pay for legal services. You can pay an hourly rate for work done, a yearly retainer, or a contingency fee. Contingency fees will normally only come into play with a lawsuit, in which the lawyer gets a percentage of the settlement. They will not apply for normal, day-to-day legal work. With a yearly retainer, you pay the lawyer a fixed fee, which covers as much or as little work as you have him or her do in the course of the year. If you don't utilize the services very much, it may not be an equitable arrangement for you; if you use the services constantly, it may not be an equitable arrangement for the attorney. If you pay an hourly rate, you pay only for work the lawyer actually does. For most small businesses, this is probably the most equitable arrangement.

Another method of paying for legal services is through menu pricing. Some attorneys offer common legal services at fixed prices. For example, the lawyer might charge $550 to set up a corporation or $25 to write and send a collection letter with one follow-up telephone call.

Once you've chosen your attorney, work closely with him or her, especially in the start-up phases of your business. Follow his or her advice, but remember that the responsibility for any final decision rests with you. Your attorney only makes recommendations and gives advice; you have the decision-making power. But before you make the decision, discuss all of the plusses and minuses of the matter. Make sure you have all the information you need to make a prudent and responsible decision.

Have your lawyer review all contracts and documents before you sign them. This is especially true in the case of leases. If you are purchasing an existing business or a franchise, get your attorney involved right from the start.

Before you start, however, go the library and read a couple of good, current business law books. Do some homework and at least learn some of the concepts. When you talk to your lawyer, it costs you money. Don't waste that money by having him or her educate you in the basic legal concepts of business. Let your lawyer earn his or her fee by doing substantive work for you.

BECOMING A LEGAL ENTITY

Before you open, your business must become a legal entity. That means it must be registered with the state, and sometimes with the locality, as a legally established business. Fictitious name statutes, in force in most states and in many municipalities, require that you register all fictitious names. A fictitious name is the trade name you use for your business, usually anything other than your real name. For example, if your name is Joan Jones and you operate as "Joan Jones Skin Care Salon," you may not need to register the name. If you operate as "Skin Care By Joan," however, that is a fictitious name and must be registered.

The registration procedure is relatively simple, normally requiring that you file registration papers with the state's office of the Secretary of State and, in some areas, with the local municipality. It is usually also necessary to publish notice of the fictitious name in one or more local newspapers to make sure there is no conflict with another business that has already registered the same name.

BUSINESS AND PROFESSIONAL LICENSES

As discussed in the previous chapter, government bodies require businesses to acquire licenses for two reasons—to raise revenues and to regulate the business operation in order to assure public safety.

To open your business, you will need a number of licenses from the state and from the community in which your salon is located. Standard business licenses that apply to all businesses, regardless of type, are relatively easy to obtain by filing with the proper authority and paying any fees. In addition, you will need a salon license issued by the state board of cosmetology, and will require an inspection by a board representative. The standard business licenses are examples of revenue raising licenses. The board license is an example of a regulatory license.

State and local licensing laws vary widely across the country. The exact licenses you will need for your business depend on where it is located. Your attorney should be able to tell you exactly which business licenses you need and should be able to file the necessary paperwork. In addition, you can get information from your state commerce department, your county courthouse, and your municipal city hall. Contact your state board of cosmetology for the specific salon licenses you will need. And make sure you and your employees have all individual professional licenses in order, as well.

Don't take the various licensing requirements lightly. Failure to obtain the licenses you need can result in severe penalties and in the closure of your salon. Make sure your salon is properly licensed and the licenses are on display, as required by the licensing authority. Renew the licenses promptly. Don't let them lapse because you've forgotten to send in the renewal fees and paperwork.

CODES AND PERMITS

Licenses are not your only concern. You also have to comply with various zoning regulations and building codes. Zoning ordinances are very important. They regulate the use of land and specify what kind of business, if any, may be conducted in a given location. They can also place physical limits on your business facilities, such as the size, location, and type of signage you may have, the exterior lighting fixtures you must install, and the size and composition of any parking facilities you utilize.

Check with your local zoning commission to get the latest regulations for your business location before you establish the salon. If you open your salon in an area where such a business is not allowed, the zoning commission can shut you down. In addition, find out the future zoning plans for the area for these can affect your planning. For example, if you've chosen the site because the traffic flow past the salon is good, and plans call for a highway overpass to be built that will drastically alter the traffic patterns, that might affect your decision to open there.

If you are buying an existing salon, don't assume that it meets the zoning requirements. It may not, and if it doesn't, you are the one who will be stuck with the consequences. Check for proper zoning compliance before you make the deal.

If your area is not zoned for a salon business, you can apply for a variance. A variance is an exception to zoning ordinances in an area and allows for nonconforming use of the land. Keep in mind, however, that zoning commissions grant variances sparingly, so don't count on getting one unless you have compelling reasons why it should be granted.

In addition to the zoning ordinances, you will also have to comply with all of the codes in effect in your community. These are designed to assure public safety by making sure your business meets minimum standards for the physical facilities. Fire codes specify the level of fire protection you need, including the number and location of exits, where you should have fire extinguishers, and whether you need to have sprinklers installed. Plumbing codes make sure you have adequate water and sewer facilities and that your restroom facilities meet standards. Electrical codes make sure your electrical service and wiring is adequate to the loads placed on them. Other building codes cover the structural soundness of the building you occupy.

Your salon will be inspected by representatives of the various code authorities to make sure you are in compliance. You will have to undergo an initial inspection when you open, then undergo periodic inspections as long as your business is in operation. Again, if you fall short of any of the code provisions, these representatives have the power to assess fines or to close the business.

Before beginning work on expansions and alterations, you must get the appropriate permits from the relevant code authority. A permit grants permission to proceed with the alteration as long as you comply with the code provisions. For example, if you decided to have new electrical wiring put in the salon, you would first have to get a permit from the building code authority, who would then inspect the finished job to make sure it met code standards.

Usually, the tradespeople you hire to make the alterations, in this example a licensed electrical contractor, will secure the necessary permits. If you decide to do the job yourself, you will have to get the permit. But the electrical code authority will want to know your qualifications to do the job safely and adequately.

If you plan on making a major expansion of your building, you will also have to check with the zoning commission to make sure the zoning ordinances allow such an expansion. Then, if it is allowed, you will have to acquire the necessary building permits. The contractor you hire will be able to help you through the paperwork.

CONTRACTS

A contract is a legally binding agreement between two or more parties. Once made, all parties must abide by the provisions of the contract, unless the parties agree to changes in the provisions. A contract carries the force of law and can be enforced by the courts.

Contracts may be written or verbal, although verbal contracts are harder to enforce, since it often comes down to one party's word against the other's. They may also be implied, so an oral promise given to someone may be held to be a legal contract. As discussed in chapter 10, that's why you must be careful what you promise to a prospective employee.

In the course of running your business, you will negotiate many different contracts. The key word is negotiate. Don't settle for less than you can reasonably accept in any contract; make sure all provisions are in writing, and don't accept any verbal promises. Have your attorney review all but the most simple contracts before you sign. Once you sign, you are bound by the provisions of the contract, whether or not they are in your favor.

The most important contract you will negotiate for your business is the lease on the property you occupy. Unlike residential leases, which offer legal protection to the lessee in most states, commercial leases offer no such legal protection. Most commercial leases are drawn up by the lessor's attorney to protect the lessor, so what you negotiate for and agree to is what you get.

Examine the terms of the lease carefully. Make sure it contains all of the provisions that are necessary for the conduct of your business, and make sure they are spelled out so there is no ambiguity. The terms of a commercial lease go far beyond the duration and the amount of rent. You must also consider a number of other factors. Do you have an option to renew the lease under favorable terms? Who pays for repairs, you or the owner? If the building is rendered unuse-able because of fire or other natural disaster, do you still pay rent? Who pays for property insurance? Who pays for taxes and utilities? Will you be reimbursed if you make improvements to the building?

What restrictions on the operation of your business are contained in the lease? Does it specify the hours or the days you can open? Are there restrictions on the type or location of signage? Are parking spaces included in the lease? Do you have use of the entire building, such as the basement or other storage areas, or are you restricted to the working areas of the salon? Who besides you has access to the building? Can the owner enter your salon while it is closed?

If you have a dispute with the owner, how will it be settled? Is there a clause in the lease that requires you go to arbitration, or will you have to go to court? Under what conditions can the owner cancel the lease? Under what conditions can you cancel the lease? What penalty will you incur if you have to cancel the lease early?

Be especially careful with lease arrangements when you are pur-chasing an existing salon. Don't assume that the current salon owner's lease will apply to you. Find out in advance whether the building owner will assign the lease in force or you will have to negotiate a new lease. If you have to negotiate a new lease, secure an agreement with the building owner before you sign an agreement to buy the business. If possible, make the sale of the business contingent on assumption of the existing lease. That shifts the burden of lease negotiation back to the seller, who already has a relationship with the landlord.

If you are buying the property in which you will establish your salon, you are still entering into a contract with the owner of the building. Once you sign the contract of sale, it is no less binding than a lease contract. Before signing, have your attorney review the contract. Remember, you are making two separate transactions. One is buying a business, the other is buying a property. Keep them separate.

Leases are not the only contracts you'll enter into. Virtually any agreement you make can be considered a contract in one way or another. When you get a business loan from the bank, you sign a con-tract. If you purchase Yellow Pages advertising, you have a contract with the telephone company. Even your telephone service and other utilities are, in effect, contracts. The point is to be aware of contractual obligations. Don't make agreements lightly. Think about what you're signing before you put your name on the line.

LIABILITIES AND RISK MANAGEMENT

Anytime you enter into a business venture, you assume some measure of risk, which may damage or destroy your business. Natural disasters, fires, theft, and flood can all hurt your salon. Other disasters, such as accidents and injuries, can incur liabilities on your part that could lead to lawsuits that would also hurt your salon.

You have negotiated your contractual liabilities and should be well aware of them. But you face noncontractual liabilities, as well. When you open your doors for business, you become responsible for the safety of your employees and clients. If someone is injured in your salon, you could be held liable for medical costs and other damages. Likewise, if one of your estheticians gives a client a facial and the client develops a rash, you could face a malpractice suit. You must take steps to reduce risk and protect yourself and your business as well as you can.

Some steps are obvious. Reduce risk of injury in your salon by practicing good housekeeping and keeping the facilities in good repair. Doing so may not eliminate the possibility of someone getting injured on your premises, but it can help you avoid charges of negligence.

Malpractice is harder to guard against. Here, one of the keys is technicians' training. Another is to establish sound, practical salon procedures that you and your employees follow to the letter. Use common sense and your best professional judgment when dealing with clients. Adhere to established industry procedures for all services and follow manufacturers' instructions on all products. For example, if everyone in the industry heats paraffin baths to 135 degrees, don't heat yours to 200 degrees because you think it might do a better, faster job. If the manufacturer of the facial mask you use says to leave it on for twenty minutes, don't leave it on for an hour because you think you'll get a better result.

Conduct patch tests when it is prudent to do so, especially when working with new clients. Have clients sign release forms when performing any services from which there may be adverse effects. Prudence dictates that you refuse to perform a service when you feel it may injure the client, even though the client may insist. For example, consider the client who wants an algae pack treatment. After examining his or her medical history, you find the client is allergic to shellfish and will probably develop a rash from the treatment. Carefully and fully explain the facts to the client, and point out the probable consequences. If he or she insists on going ahead anyway, you have to decide whether to do the procedure. Bear in mind that either way, you may lose the client. However, it is probably better to lose a client because you refused the service than because you went ahead and damaged his or her skin.

Remember you are the professional and ostensibly the expert in the field. Even if the client signs a release and takes responsibility for any damage, if he or she later sues you, the courts may hold that the release is invalid because your expertise should have taken precedence and you went ahead with the procedure, even though you knew there was a high probability of damage to the skin.

How do you protect yourself? Unfortunately, it is impossible to protect yourself and your business against every risk, especially malpractice suits. In this age, anybody can sue anyone for anything at anytime. Your best defense may be to show you were not negligent and followed all the rules. You can further protect yourself by carrying adequate insurance coverage.

INSURANCE

Insurance is a basic part of risk management. In essence, it is a sharing of the risk between two parties, the insurer and the insured. You purchase a policy from an insurance company that, for a fee, will protect you from loss if the insured event occurs. A policy is a legal contract that consists of a number of elements—an offer, acceptance, consideration, legal purpose, and insurable interest. You make an offer when you apply for the policy and make a payment. The insurance company accepts the offer when it cashes your check and issues the policy. Consideration is an exchange of promises; that is, you agree to pay the premiums and the insurance company agrees to pay the damages. For the contract to be valid, the insurance must be for a legal purpose and you must have an insurable interest in the insured item. For example, you can insure your salon but not your competitor's. And there must be no misrepresentation of material facts; that is, you have told the truth on the application, at least about everything that is relevant to the insurance coverage.

CHECKLIST 7-2
INSURANCE COVERAGE

Types of insurance to consider:

1. Casualty insurance protects you against physical damage.
    A. Fire insurance.
    B. Business interruption insurance.
    C. Glass and sign insurance.
    D. Automobile insurance.
2. Liability insurance protects you against lawsuits.
    A. Accident and negligence insurance.
    B. Employee theft and misconduct insurance.
    C. Malpractice insurance.
3. Life, health, and disability insurance protects you or your survivors from loss due to death or illness.

Insurance is governed by state regulations through the state insurance commission. However, each state has its own laws, so check with a qualified insurance representative in your state. Discuss your insurance needs with your attorney, as well. If you have specific questions about insurance regulations, call your state insurance commission.

There are many different kinds of insurance, usually covering some aspect of casualty; liability; or life, health, and disability. You can buy an insurance policy to cover virtually any form of risk. Some policies are vital for your business regardless of circumstances; some are useful under certain circumstances.

Casualty Insurance Policies

Casualty insurance covers you against physical damage from such things as fire, floods, earthquakes, and natural disasters. Fire insurance covers you in the event of damage due to fire, whether caused by accident, by lightning, or by intention. Good fire insurance coverage is vital to your business.

Business interruption insurance covers your salon from losses as a result of a major disaster, such as a hurricane or earthquake, that closes your business down. It may also protect you from lost business caused by fire or vandalism. This type of insurance can be expensive. Base your decision on the likelihood of such disasters occurring in your area.

Glass and sign insurance are specific policies that cover your plate glass windows and your signs. Plate glass and signs, especially neon or internally illuminated signs, are expensive to replace. These policies are relatively inexpensive and can save you money if you have to replace the items.

Auto insurance covers both casualty and liability. The collision part of the policy pays for damages incurred to your vehicle when involved in an accident. Comprehensive insurance covers physical damage not covered by the collision insurance. The liability part protects you from damages in the event of your negligence. This insurance may not be applicable to the salon, unless you operate a vehicle for some business reason connected with the salon. Keep in mind, however, that if you send an employee on an errand by car, and he or she is involved in an accident, you could be held liable for damages. Consider buying auto insurance if you regularly utilize a vehicle in the business.

Liability Insurance Policies

Liability insurance protects you from damages and lawsuits for acts in which you were negligent or could be held at fault. Basic liability insurance is vital to your business. It covers you, for example, if a client slips and falls in your salon and gets hurt. Tenant's and owner's insurance covers you for basic liability arising from the use or maintenance of the building and grounds, for example, if a passerby trips and falls on the sidewalk outside your building. This is also vital coverage.

Employee theft and misconduct insurance covers the salon against the actions of your workers and will reimburse you for losses if, for example, your receptionist runs off with the day's receipts or if your employee gets into an argument with a client and punches him or her. The need for this type of insurance varies with the quality of your staff and how much you trust them.

Malpractice insurance covers you from damages incurred as a result of your professional practices. If a client develops a skin allergy as a result of a facial, for example, you will be protected from monetary losses. Your reputation will still suffer, however. In this day and age, some form of malpractice insurance is absolutely necessary.

Life, Health, and Disability Insurance Policies

Life insurance protects your business from the consequences of the death of a partner or yourself. What happens to your business if you or a partner dies? Such an event could force you, your heirs, or your partners to sell the business or be faced with severe tax consequences. Life insurance can protect the business from this, so you should have some coverage here.

Health and disability insurance pays all or part of the hospital and doctor bills you incur as a result of illness or accident. Major medical insurance pays for catastrophic illness. Lost income insurance makes up for the income you lose while unable to work. Some form of health and disability insurance is important for you. You may also want to offer this insurance coverage to your employees as part of their benefits package. There are many suppliers of health and disability insurance, offering a broad array of group plans. You can choose to pick up the entire cost for your employees, or as is more commonly the case, have them pay for part of the coverage.

DETERMINING YOUR INSURANCE COVERAGE

Insurance can be expensive. If you bought a policy to protect you against every possible contingency, you would probably go bankrupt. You can't afford to buy more than you need and you can't afford not to buy enough to ensure the survival of your business. You want to buy coverage that will give you what you really need at a price that is acceptable to your bottom line—and no more.

The first step in determining how much and what kind of insurance you need is to assess your level of risk. Think about the risks you might face, and consider only those that have some probability of occurring. Don't worry about everything that could possibly happen. For example, if your salon is located in an area that hasn't had an earthquake in the past three hundred years, it's not very probable you'll have to worry about that risk. Don't limit your thinking to casualty risks. Consider risks stemming from liability and life, as well.

Make a list of those risks, then consider the consequences of such an event. Give priority to those consequences that most affect the survivability of your salon. Thus, you might give more weight to a fire that guts your building and closes your business for an extended time than you would to a storm that shatters your plate glass window and closes you for only a few hours.

Now consider the monetary value of the consequences. An event that closes your salon permanently could wipe you out. Settling with an irate client could cost you only a few hundred dollars. (Or much more, depending on the level of injury he or she suffered.) Then decide how much of that monetary risk you are willing to assume yourself and how much you want to share with the insurer. Also consider what alternatives you can take, either to reduce the level of risk or to reduce the cost of insurance, for example by adding a sprinkler system in the salon to reduce the possibility of losses from fire or to reduce the fire insurance premiums. Also, how high do you want to set the deductibles? The higher your deductible, the amount of risk you pay for before the insurance coverage starts, the lower the premiums.

Also, be aware of insurance you are required to have. If you have a bank loan, for example, the bank may require you to have basic life and business insurance coverage. The state may require you to carry workers' compensation insurance. Your lease may require that you carry a certain level of tenant's insurance.

Then set your budget for insurance. Like any expense, you must budget for insurance costs. Decide how much you're willing to pay for coverage and allow for it in your financial planning.

CHOOSING AN INSURANCE SOURCE

Once you have considered your needs, know your insurance requirements, and have a budget established, shop for the best coverage. You have a choice of dealing either with an independent insurance broker or with an insurance company agent. Brokers represent a number of different companies and may be able to find policies that fill a broader range of your requirements. A company agent, on the other hand, may be able to better tailor the policies offered by his or her company to your specific needs. Also, many trade associations offer various insurance packages specially designed for the salon business that include malpractice coverage as well as a number of health and hospitalization plans. Look into these plans, as well.

Talk to your peers in the industry as well as to other business people to get recommendations. Choose your insurance agent with the same careful investigation you used to pick your attorney, your accountant, your banker, and other advisors. Talk to several agents with several insurance companies. Make sure you communicate your needs to the agents, then make sure they discuss insurance coverage based on your needs and not on what they have to sell. Ask questions, and be sure you understand all of the aspects of the insurance coverage they suggest. Be wary of standardized insurance packages that many companies may offer. You need, and should demand, insurance coverage tailored to your specific needs.

Get quotes on the various insurance coverages and compare them. Pick what best suits your needs and budget. As with any service, don't base your decision only on price. With insurance, service and the willingness of the agent to work with you is important. If you have questions about the reputation or reliability of the insurance company or companies you are considering, check with your state insurance commission.

SUMMARY

There is far more to starting a salon than just opening the doors for business. You must be aware of and comply with all of the legal requirements necessary to your business. These include becoming a legal entity by registering with the state, obtaining all of the licenses and permits you will need, and making yourself familiar with the applicable laws. To do these things safely and properly, you should have legal representation. Hire a competent attorney early in your planning stage, then work closely with him or her.

In the course of running your business, you will negotiate many contracts. It is important to remember that a contract is a legally binding agreement. Once you have signed it, you are bound by its terms, so be careful. Make sure you understand all the provisions of any contract, and have your attorney review all contracts before you sign.

Risk is a part of any business. For your own protection, you must be aware of the risks you face and take steps to minimize them. One of the key risks you face in your salon is malpractice. Make sure you know what you're doing with any service, and follow sound industry practices. When you use a product, always follow the manufacturer's directions.

One way to protect yourself is to get insurance coverage. There are a number of different insurance policies that can help protect you against a variety of hazards. Discuss your needs with a competent insurance agent.

CAPITALIZATION AND FINANCING

C H A P T E R
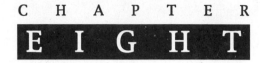

Nothing will be so important to the start up of your salon as having sufficient capital; that is, enough money to open your doors for business and to keep your salon running for at least a year with little or no income. Insufficient capital is perhaps the most common reason that businesses fail. They just don't have enough cash to stay open and keep going. They don't have the means to weather the inevitable problems and unexpected expenses that arise in the early start-up phase of the business. Very early in your planning cycle, you should ask yourself four basic questions: How much money do I need to open the business? How much money will I need to run the business during my first year of operation? How much of that money do I have? Where am I going to get the rest of the money I need?

To help you answer these questions, you should seek the counsel of two persons who will be extremely important to your business success—your accountant and your banker. Your accountant will help you determine your capital requirements and will help you prepare the documentation you need to present to the bank to get financing. Your banker will help you get the funds to finance those capital needs. A word of caution here, though. Be careful when discussing your business with a banker. To get counseling, you have to expose your limitations and shortcomings. You should never discuss these with someone from whom you may want to borrow funds.

CHECKLIST 8-1
CHOOSING AN ACCOUNTANT

When choosing an accountant:

1. Get recommendations.
2. Look for a small accounting firm.
3. Look for a certified public accountant.
4. Interview candidates thoroughly.
5. Determine expertise in small business affairs.
6. Discuss your needs and requirements.
7. Discuss fee structure.
8. Check references.

CHOOSING AN ACCOUNTANT

Once you've made the decision to open your salon, one of the first steps you should take is to find and hire a good accountant. He or she will have a profound effect on your business, so take your time, interview several candidates, and choose wisely. Your accountant is an independent contractor that you pay only for time and services rendered. He or she is not an employee. Hire the best accountant you can. Don't try to save a few dollars here. A good accountant should be able to save you much more than he or she charges you for services rendered.

Get recommendations from friends, bankers, other small business managers, and other salon owners. Look for a small accounting firm that has experience in working with small businesses and has a reputation for integrity. A small firm will generally offer more personalized service at lower prices than large accounting firms. Also, with a small firm, you will probably work with the same accountant and be better able to establish a one-on-one business relationship. The accountant should be a certified public accountant, a licensed professional who has passed a rigorous examination and has demonstrated expertise in the field.

Interview each candidate carefully. Ask about his or her expertise, experience with small business, and background. Ask about specific experience in working with salons. How many clients does the firm have, and how much time is allocated to each? Will the candidate do the actual work, or will it be delegated to someone else in the firm? How many hours does the candidate feel will be necessary to handle your accounting needs? Is he or she willing to spend the time necessary at the start to help you set up your accounting and bookkeeping systems and to monitor their effectiveness?

Discuss the fee structure. How much will services cost and what will the price include? Is the retainer all-inclusive or will you pay extra for financial reports and for tax services? What additional services are you likely to need that are not included in the retainer?

Get references from the candidates and check a number of them at random. Also, consider how you feel about the candidates. Which are you most comfortable with? Who gives you a feeling of confidence? Who seems more in line with your needs and ideas? Which was best able to explain accounting concepts to your satisfaction and understanding? Consider all these things, then make your choice, but choose prudently. You can, of course, always change accountants if you're not getting the service you need, but changing can be difficult and confusing.

CHOOSING A BANK

Another important step you should take early in your planning cycle is to establish a relationship with a bank. Choose your bank with the same care you choose your accountant and attorney. Like those people, your bank can be a help to your business.

A bank is a company that is chartered by the federal government or by the state in which it operates to conduct a broad range of financial activities, including accepting deposits, making loans and investments, and providing financial services such as advice and trust management. Think of a bank as a business, like yours, but whose product is money. Banks make money through interest-bearing loans and investments. They acquire much of the funds used to make these loans and investments by accepting money from clients, which is deposited into checking accounts and accounts on which the banks pay interest, such as Money Market accounts, NOW and Super-NOW accounts, Certificates of Deposit, and other savings accounts.

There are many types of commercial and noncommercial banks. Commercial banks include the Federal Reserve banks, investment and mortgage banks, and nationally and state chartered banks, which primarily service the needs of business. Noncommercial banks include the thrift institutions, such as credit unions and savings and loan institutions, which primarily service the needs of consumers. However, there is a broad overlap of functions, as many commercial banks also provide services for consumers and many thrift institutions also service business accounts. Most offer commercial and consumer loans as well as a wide variety of checking and savings accounts for businesses and consumers. Most savings and loan institutions, savings banks, and credit unions are excluded by their charters from making business loans.

You will need at least two accounts for your business—a checking account and a business savings account. You will use your checking account to pay your bills, payrolls, and other expenses, but these accounts seldom draw interest, so you don't want to keep any more money in a checking account than you need to cover your expenses. For the excess, you should have an interest-bearing business savings account of some type. The idea is to have your idle money working for you. Whatever type of account you open, however, make sure you have the flexiblity to transfer funds from that account to your checking account whenever you need the money. Some savings accounts offer higher interest rates, but your money is frozen for a definite time period. In this case, you want to sacrifice interest rate for liquidity.

If you will accept credit cards from your clients, i.e. MasterCard, Visa, American Express, or Diner's Club, make sure the bank will handle those transactions, too.

You may also want to open an IRA (Individual Retirement Account) both for your future and as a tax shelter. You can contribute money to an IRA account on a pre-tax basis, but you have limited access to that money. If you withdraw it before a specified age, you'll have to pay tax and penalties on the funds.

Choose your bank in much the same way you chose your accountant. Look for a small to midsize commercial bank or thrift institution, preferably with a branch in the same neighborhood as your salon. The bank should have experience in working with small businesses and should be able to offer you a complete range of services. Interview officials at a number of banks. Let them know what you need and expect and find out what they're willing to do for you. What services do they offer? Do they make loans to small busi-nesses? Will you have a specific person in the bank you can work with, or will you be dealing with a different person each time? What recommendations can they make about your requirements? Compare the banks and see which one best meets your needs. Then consider how you feel about the various banks. Which one made you most comfortable? Which seemed most willing to work with you? In which were you most confident? You are looking for a long term rela-tionship with the bank, so the chemistry between you and the people you'll be working with there is important.

Once you've chosen the bank, open your business accounts. You might also want to switch your personal accounts there, as well. At some point, you will be looking for a business loan from them. The more business you give them and the better they get to know you and value you as a customer, the more likely you are to get the loan. Be aware, though, that just because you have a number of accounts with that bank, there's no guarantee that your loan will be approved. But your accounts are a significant bargaining chip for you, either with your bank or with another.

DETERMINE YOUR CAPITAL REQUIREMENTS

Your next step is to determine your capital requirements. How much money do you need to open your salon and how much do you need to keep it in operation for at least a year? This information should be contained in the financial elements of your business plan, which con-cern the tangible physical aspects of your business, i. e., location, equipment, supplies, and services you have to buy or lease. You develop this information by establishing your preliminary budget.

As discussed in Chapter 2, your first budget consideration is the physical facility you will utilize. Are you renting the building or buying it? Consider the monthly rent or mortgage payment including, in the case of rented facilities, additional rents and security deposits or, in the case of a building you own, property taxes and escrow payments.

Also, as part of your physical facilities budget, you will have to consider what it will cost to make the building suitable for your use, in terms of decoration and renovation. And don't forget your signage

CHECKLIST 8-2
DETERMINING CAPITAL REQUIREMENTS

Factors in determining capital requirements:

1. Physical facilities
   A. Building—lease or purchase
   B. Decoration and renovation
   C. Utilities
2. Capital equipment
   A. Equipment to perform services
   B. Equipment for administration
3. Noncapital equipment and supplies
4. Staffing needs
   A. Number and type of employees
   B. Salary requirements
   C. Benefits and other employee costs
5. Purchased services
   A. Accounting and bookkeeping
   B. Legal services
   C. Towel and laundry services
   D. Telephone service
6. License and permit fees
7. Advertising and promotion

needs. These are one-time costs. However, don't forget to budget monthly costs for utilities, and water and sewer rents.

Next, consider your capital equipment requirements, i.e. those pieces of machinery or apparatus necessary to perform the services you want to provide as well as equipment for the administrative aspects of the business. Also consider your noncapital equipment requirements, i.e. those items that have a shorter life span and can be deducted fully in the purchase year as a business expense. Don't forget other significant one-time expenses, such as graphic design fees for logos, layouts for business cards, and brochures. Printing costs can be a significant start-up expense.

Decide what and how much equipment you will need and whether you will purchase or lease the equipment. Determine your equipment costs or lease payments as part of your budget. Supplies come next. You will need a minimum of supplies, including consumable and reusable items, just to get started. Estimate your needs for consumable and disposable items for at least one month, and base your figure on that cost. Then add the costs for a reasonable supply of the reusable items.

You must also allow for your staffing needs. Determine the minimum number and type of employees you will need to start, including yourself and any working partners. How much are you going to pay these people? Where are you going to get the money to pay them? Don't forget to include your own salary requirements. Estimated salaries are not the only expense to consider. You will also have to allow for benefits and other employee costs, such as workers' compensation and Social Security payments.

You must also consider services you will purchase. These may include accounting, bookkeeping, and legal services as well as towel and laundry services. Don't forget telephone services. Add in, also, any fees you may be required to pay, such as licensing fees and fictitious name registrations. Also allow some preliminary expenses for advertising and promotion. At the least, you should allow for telephone directory advertisements and local newspaper ads.

Develop your preliminary budgets from the figures you've established for each of these categories. You need two budgets. The start-up budget lists all of the one-time expenses you will incur in opening your salon. The preliminary operating budget lists your estimated recurring expenses to keep the business going. The total of the two budgets will be the amount of money you will need to get your business started and keep it in operation for the first year. Be careful when you establish these preliminary budgets. Unless you are buying an already established salon, you won't have a business history to draw cost data from, so you will have to make the best estimates you can, especially with the preliminary operating budget. But make the figures as accurate as you can. Don't underestimate your needs. Your start-up will probably require more cash than you think.

SOURCES OF CAPITAL

Once you know how much money it will take to establish your salon, you have to consider where the money will come from and when you will need it. There are only two basic sources of money for your venture—your own resources or other people's resources.

CHECKLIST 8-3
SOURCES OF CAPITAL

1. Personal Sources
   A. Savings
   B. Other assets
   C. Other sources of income
   D. Personal loans
      1. From banks and finance companies
      2. From credit cards
      3. From friends and relatives
2. Business Sources
   A. Equity capital
      1. Partners
      2. Sale of shares
      3. Small Business Investment Companies
      4. Venture capitalists
      5. Special minority programs
   B. Debt capital
      1. Business loans
         a. From commercial banks and finance companies
         b. From the Small Business Administration
         c. Trade credit
         d. Leasing

Personal Sources of Financing

Your first resource should be yourself. You should be able to utilize your own savings and assets or draw from personal resources to finance a good portion of your salon. The more of your own funds you can invest, the less you'll need from other sources and the more readily banks and other lenders will be willing to lend to you. Look at all of your personal assets first. How much money do you have? What is the source of that money? Is it from savings accounts or certificates of deposit? From the sale of other assets such as stocks and bonds? From other sources of income, such as another job or royalties? How much of your own money are you willing or able to provide? If you have partners, how much will they provide, and what are the sources of their contributions to the business?

In conjunction with your accountant, develop a financial statement that lists your personal assets and liabilities. The statement should show any and all sources of income, plus assets such as equity in your home, savings, stocks, and bonds. It should also list your personal debts, such as mortgages, credit card payments, and auto loans. Once you know your financial situation, you'll know how much of your own funds you can allocate to your business. You'll then decide how much of that money you are willing to invest in your salon. It should be as much as you can afford. After all, if you're not willing to take a chance on your salon, why should other people?

Now you should determine how much you can raise from personal sources. Will you borrow from friends or family, or will you seek personal loans from banks, credit unions, or finance companies? Will you get an equity loan on property you own? Will you utilize cash advances on credit cards? If you borrow money, how will you pay it back? What terms will you require? What will you offer as collateral?

Borrowing from friends and family has advantages and disadvantages. It is often easier to borrow from these sources. Their requirements will certainly be less stringent than those of a bank or finance company, and the repayment terms will usually be more agreeable. However, the resources of your friends and family may be more limited than those of a bank, and they may not have enough to cover your needs. Also, remember that you are still borrowing money that will have to be repaid at some point. Even though the source is friends or family, there should be a written loan agreement, with interest and repayment terms clearly listed. Without such an agreement, the IRS may consider the money to be a gift rather than a loan and hit your backers with a hefty tax bill.

When you're first starting in business, you may find it easier to obtain personal loans from banks, credit unions, or finance companies than to obtain business loans, even from these same sources. You will generally require some form of collateral, that is real or personal property you pledge to insure payment of the loan. If you default, the lender can take the property to satisfy the debt. While easier to obtain, personal loans have the disadvantage that they will be considered among your liabilities if you apply for a business loan from a bank.

You might also consider using credit cards, especially to purchase equipment or supplies. Keep in mind, however, that interest rates on credit card loans and most personal loans may be higher than on comparable business loans. In addition, interest payments for personal loans are not deductible on your income tax, even if the money was used for business purposes.

Business Sources of Financing

Once you have exhausted your own personal resources, whether your own assets or personal loans, there are two forms of capital you can seek. One is debt capital; the other is equity capital. Debt capital consists of borrowed money, regardless of the source. It is money normally borrowed for relatively short term periods and must be repaid. It does not affect ownership of the business. The people who advance the money do not become owners, but they receive a return on their money through interest paid on the loan.

Equity capital consists of money invested in the business by investors in exchange for a share of ownership in the business. In this case, the people who put up the money become part owners of the business. While this money does not have to be repaid, the investors will expect to receive a share of the profits in the form of dividends. They receive a return on their money through the appreciation in the value of the business. The personal funds you put into your business are your equity capital.

SOURCES OF DEBT CAPITAL

There are a number of possible sources of debt capital. These include commercial bank loans, SBA loans or guarantees, commercial finance companies, trade credit, and leasing. Each offers a number of advantages and disadvantages, but none should be overlooked when you need money for your salon.

Commercial Bank Loans

The most common form of debt capital is a business loan from a commercial bank. Depending on the economic climate at the time you apply for a business loan, your chances of having it approved vary from very easy to almost impossible, especially if you are just starting your salon. Banks make their decisions based on the amount of risk they must assume. Therefore, they will look very closely at your credit history, your probability of business success, and your ability to pay back the loan. The more information you can provide to your banker, the better your chances of receiving the loan. Be open and honest and provide all the data, especially financial information, he or she requests, and be prepared to document the information. At a minimum, you will have to provide the following information:

- *A full description of your salon:* Provide name, address, telephone number, the services you provide, and the demographics of the clients you serve.
- *How much money you want to borrow and what you want to use it for:* Ask for all the money you will need and be specific about how you'll spend it.
- *How you plan to repay the loan:* Suggest a payment schedule that fits your needs, and provide financial information that shows the banker where the money will come from. These include profit and loss statements and cash flow statements for at least the past three years, if you have been in business that long. If you are just starting in business, provide your best forecasts, as prepared by you and your accountant.
- *Your business plan:* Your written business plan, as discussed in Chapter 2, will provide much of the information your banker will need.
- *Personal information:* Provide financial data, such as your personal assets and liabilities, as well as information about your experience and ability to conduct your salon business. Include personal and professional references, if you have them.
- *Business assets you can pledge as collateral:* Just as personal assets provide collateral for a personal loan, your business assets can be used as collateral for a commercial loan. These business assets generally take the form of accounts receivable, inventory, or equipment. Accounts receivable are monies owed to you by clients. In effect, you are pledging the income from sales you've already made but haven't yet collected. Inventory covers goods that have already been made or stocked but haven't yet been sold, or the raw materials used to make the goods.

Inventory and accounts receivable are more suitable for a manufacturing or retail business than a service business like a salon. Most esthetics salons operate by selling skin care and other beauty services on a cash or credit card basis. You will not have any accounts receivable unless you offer your services on credit, for which you bill and collect from your clients. Nor do most salons manufacture products or stock large amounts of goods for retail sale. Your inventory will be limited to those items you use in the salon or offer for retail sale as an adjunct to your salon service activities. You will probably never have enough inventory or accounts receivable to be acceptable to a bank as collateral. Nor will most banks consider your salon inventory or equipment as collateral for a start-up loan. Usually, they will consider only assets that can be sold reasonably quickly, such as vehicles and buildings. Unless you own the building in which your salon is located, the only business asset you will be able to offer as collateral is your equipment, and that may not be acceptable to the bank.

Be prepared to offer personal guarantees; that is, pledge personal assets as collateral or have one or more cosigners for the loan. A cosigner, or guarantor, is a third party to the transaction who provides a guarantee that the loan will be repaid. If you default, the bank can collect from the third party.

There are a number of types of business, or commercial, loans. The majority of commercial loans are short-term and run for a period ranging from thirty to ninety days, although some extend to one year. They are usually repaid in a lump sum, consisting of both principal and interest, at the end of the loan period. These short-term loans are usually made to provide working capital, i.e. money to purchase supplies or to take advantage of an especially good deal on equipment or other materials. If your salon has a good credit history, you may be able to get an unsecured short-term loan, although the bank may require your personal guarantee. Otherwise, you'll have to secure the loan through collateral.

Intermediate term loans run from one to five years and are similar to short-term loans, except for the payment schedule. These loans generally require that periodic payments be made, i. e. monthly, quarterly, semi-annually, or annually. Intermediate term loans are usually made to provide money for expansion or to purchase an existing business. The amounts involved are generally larger than short-term loans. They are seldom unsecured, and collateral is almost always required.

Long-term loans extend beyond five years and are usually for the purchase of real estate or facilities. Like mortgages, they are secured by real property. These loans generally are for large amounts of money and require periodic payments.

Lines of credit are another form of business loan. A line of credit is a pre-arranged amount of money that is kept in the bank and may be borrowed against as needed. You can get what amounts to a virtually automatic loan whenever you need the money, as long as you don't exceed the agreed-upon amount. Although some of these loans may be unsecured, most lines of credit for small businesses will be secured by all business assets as well as personal guarantees. They may be for one-time use, that is, as you draw on the funds, they are no longer available, even after you've paid them back. Or they may be revolving, that is, like a credit card, as you pay back the funds, the amount is again available for use. Lines of credit are short-term loans that are usually utilized for working capital requirements and repaid quickly.

Whatever type of commercial loan you acquire, you will be expected to sign a loan agreement, which will contain the terms and conditions of the loan. You may have to agree to a number of covenants, or restrictions on how you conduct your business, during the term of the loan. These covenants are for the bank's protection and provide a measure of control over your operations. They may include items such as restrictions on the amount of money you or other owners may draw as salary. They may require that you use the borrowed funds only for the purpose you stated in the application or prevent you from borrowing additional money from another source while the loan agreement is in effect.

Covenants are legally binding. If you violate one of them, the bank can declare the loan in default and demand that you pay back the entire amount immediately. So, before you sign the loan agreement, read it thoroughly, and make sure you understand all of the terms and covenants in the document. Don't sign if you disagree with a covenant. Most covenants are negotiable, but only if you negotiate before you sign. Get all agreements in writing. Don't rely on verbal promises or commitments from the banker.

SBA Loans

If you are unable to acquire a loan from a bank, you may be able to get the money from the Small Business Administration. The SBA is a federal government agency established to provide assistance and advice to small businesses. It helps them find financing and gives management and financial counsel to owners and managers. To qualify for a loan, you must meet the SBA's definition of a small business; that is, your salon must be privately owned and operated, and you must have annual gross receipts of less than $2 million. Under this definition, virtually every salon in existence qualifies. In addition, you must meet certain credit requirements, including expertise in salon operations, ability to manage on a financially sound basis, and ability to repay the loan from earnings. You must also be of good moral character.

You may be considered for an SBA loan only if you cannot obtain a loan from a bank or other commercial source and have exhausted all other avenues of financing. If you do qualify, you will most likely apply for the loan under the SBA's 7(a) Program that provides for either direct loans from the agency or for loans from a lending institution, which are then guaranteed by the SBA.

In a guaranteed loan, the money comes from the bank or other lending institution. The SBA guarantees payment for 90 percent of the money. That means if you default on the loan, 90 percent of the money will be paid to the bank by the federal government. Most SBA loans are of this type. The agency makes few direct loans.

As with other commercial loans, you will be required to provide collateral for the SBA loan. The same types of collateral, business or personal assets, are acceptable. Loan duration may not exceed ten years. Repayment of principal and interest is usually on a monthly basis. Interest rates for SBA loans are higher than commercial bank rates, usually 3/4 to 1 percent higher.

For complete information and current regulations, contact the Small Business Administration field office in your area. The telephone number will be listed in the local telephone directory.

Commercial Finance Companies

Other possible sources of debt capital are commercial finance companies that, like banks, lend money to businesses. They accept higher risk loans and, consequently, charge higher interest rates. Their credit requirements are similar to those for banks, and they offer loans on much the same terms of repayment and duration. Commercial finance companies seldom give unsecured loans. Typically, loans from these sources are guaranteed by accounts receivable, inventory, equipment, or real estate.

When it comes to collateral, you will encounter the same difficulty with a commercial finance company that you encounter with a bank, namely, no accounts receivable or inventory. You may use equipment you already have as collateral, however.

Commercial finance companies sometimes offer industrial time purchase agreements for those who purchase new equipment. In these cases, the company acts as a third party to a transaction between you and the manufacturer or wholesaler of the equipment. You purchase the equipment from the seller. The finance company gives the money to the seller. You repay the finance company for the amount of the purchase plus interest. The finance company retains ownership of the equipment as collateral until the loan is paid, although you have the use of it.

Trade Credit

Trade credit, the type of credit you may be able to get from your suppliers, does not take the form of cash, but comes in the form of more favorable payment terms for supplies and equipment. If a supplier will give you thirty to ninety days to pay for your supplies, for example, that has the same effect as borrowing that amount of money for the same period. And, there's no interest.

If you are just starting in business, you may find it difficult to get trade credit, however. A supplier is more likely to give you favorable terms after you have established a good track record as a customer. If you have good relationships with your suppliers, don't be afraid to ask for trade credit. They won't offer it to you on their own.

You may also be able to purchase equipment on a time payment plan from the manufacturer or wholesaler. This is similar to an industrial time purchase agreement discussed under commercial finance companies, except that there is no third party involved. You make payments directly to the seller. As above, the seller retains ownership of the equipment until the debt is paid. Although you will not need additional collateral, you may have to make a substantial down payment on the equipment.

Leasing

Leasing is another way to acquire equipment for your salon. It is an alternative method of financing that lets you have full use of the equipment while never owning it. There are a number of advantages to leasing. You don't have to worry about the equipment becoming obsolete. You just turn it back to the leasing company and re-lease an updated version. There are also tax advantages. The monthly lease payment is an operating expense and is fully deductible on your taxes. Equipment you own, however, must be depreciated over a fixed period of time, so you don't get the same tax benefit.

A disadvantage of leasing is that it can be more expensive over the long term. Unless you have a lease-purchase option that lets you acquire ownership of the equipment for a fee at the end of the lease agreement, you will have to lease another piece of equipment or sign a new lease agreement for the current equipment. You continue to make monthly payments. If you purchase the equipment, once it is paid for you have no further payments to make. If the equipment has a relatively short life span before it must be replaced, leasing may be preferable. On the other hand, if the equipment has a relatively long life span, it may be better to purchase it. Lease agreements generally require a substantial down payment, which usually covers security and the first few months' rent.

When you purchase new equipment, check with the manufacturer or wholesaler about lease terms. Study the pros and cons of the lease carefully, then make your choice. Discuss the arrangements with your accountant before making your decision. A lease agreement is a legal contract, and you must comply with the terms.

SOURCES OF EQUITY CAPITAL

It is possible to raise equity capital from a number of sources. These include selling full or limited partnerships, selling shares to relatives or friends, receiving funds from Small Business Investment Companies, or selling an interest in the company to venture capitalists. Whatever the source, however, remember you're selling ownership in your business and giving up some measure of control. These investors will be able to exercise some degree of direction over the management of the salon. As mentioned earlier, equity capital is for long term needs and is permanent. The investors retain ownership in your business unless you can buy the shares back from them in the future.

Partnerships

One of the most common ways of bringing equity capital into the business is by adding one or more new partners. These may be either general partners, who play a significant role in the management of the business, or limited partners, who receive shares in the profits but are not active in the day-to-day operations of the salon. (Refer to Chapter 3 for a complete description of partnerships.) Keep in mind the tax and liability options, and make sure all conditions are contained in a written partnership agreement.

Sales of Shares

If you have formed a corporation, either an S-corporation or a C-corporation, you can sell limited shares of stock to relatives and friends, as long as you don't make a public offering. Public stock offerings are complicated and expensive and are heavily regulated by the Securities and Exchange Commission. They are suitable only for large companies. As with any financial transaction, follow your accountant's counsel and have written agreements.

Small Business Investment Companies

Small Business Investment Companies (SBICs) are private firms, licensed and partially funded by the SBA, that provide equity capital to small businesses. They are not part of the Small Business Administration. These companies provide funds to small businesses, usually in return for shares of stock or other ownership rights. In some cases, they make loans to a business instead of purchasing stock. Contact your local SBA office for more information.

Venture Capital

Venture capitalists are private individuals who invest money in businesses in return for ownership equity. These investors may operate as individuals, as part of a venture capital club, or as part of a firm specializing in venture capital funding. Venture capital firms are usually only interested in larger, high-tech companies, so your chances of getting funds from one of these are slim. However, venture capital clubs or individuals may be able to provide the money you require.

Potential leads for finding venture capital may come from almost any source. Your accountant or attorney may be aware of possible investors. Don't overlook your customers, either. Some of them may be interested in providing equity capital for a share of the profits. For a directory of venture capital clubs, contact the International Venture Capital Institute in Stamford, Connecticut.

OTHER SOURCES OF FINANCING

If you are a woman or a member of a minority group, you may qualify for funding under a variety of special programs sponsored by federal and state government agencies and private groups and foundations.

Women and minority business owners are covered under the Equal Credit Opportunity Act. Under this law, a lender cannot consider your sex, race, national origin, or marital status when deciding if your loan application will be honored. If you believe you have been unlawfully denied a loan because of discrimination, contact the regulatory agency that supervises the lending institution.

The Small Business Administration's Program 8(a) makes direct loans to minorities, the socially disadvantaged, the handicapped, and Vietnam veterans who want to operate their own businesses. The SBA also administers the Minority Enterprise Small Business Investment Company program. Like SBICs, MESBICs provide equity capital or make direct loans to small business owners, but their funds are specifically earmarked for the use of minority business people. Contact your local SBA field office for more information about either of these programs. Some state government agencies also administer programs geared to minority needs. Contact your local state representative for information about programs in your state.

In addition, some private programs provide financing for women and minorities. For example, the National Association for Female Executives will lend up to $50,000 to women who meet their requirements.

Note that these government and private agencies still have quite stringent credit requirements. You must still be able to offer a sound business and financial plan and document your facts. Loans from these sources are not guaranteed. You must still do your homework.

SUMMARY

If you are going to be successful in your business, you must have adequate capital. You must have enough money to get the things you need to operate the business and to pay expenses. Lack of sufficient capital is the reason many businesses fail. To help you determine your needs and to acquire the funds, you should work with an accountant and a banker. Choose them carefully.

You need enough capital to open your salon and to keep it in operation for at least a year. Your business plan should contain this information. You need to know what physical facilities you'll need, the equipment you'll have to get, the staff you'll need, and the services you'll have to purchase. From this information, you will establish a budget.

Once you know how much money you will need, you have to determine where it will come from. There are a number of sources of capital. Part of the money will be your own—money you have in savings or in other assets, as well as money you can borrow as personal loans. Part of the money will be equity capital, coming from other people, either partners or investors, who will share in the ownership of the business. Or it may be debt capital, that is, business loans from banks or finance companies. Under some conditions, you may be able to get financing from the Small Business Administration.

FINANCIAL MANAGEMENT
AND ACCOUNTING

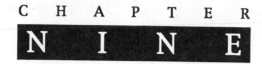

C H A P T E R
N I N E

Profit is not a dirty word. It is, or should be, the reason you're in business. If it is not, you probably shouldn't be in business for yourself. You started your own salon because you wanted more independence and more freedom to do your own thing. In short, you wanted to have the financial liberty to let you live the lifestyle you chose. To do that, your salon must make a profit.

Making a profit is no simple matter. It involves more than just counting the revenue that comes into the shop. You must also consider your expenses, your time, and your effort. It is possible to have high revenues, but have such high overhead that you are actually losing money. That's a trap you can fall into very easily.

You can avoid that trap by exercising sound financial management principles and following proper accounting procedures. These will let you control your expenses, make sure you pay no more taxes than you are obligated to pay, and keep the services you offer profitable. But you must think like a business manager, not like an esthetician. It takes time and effort to do the job properly. You have to examine all aspects of the business and keep watch over all operations, and you have to do it on a regular basis. Your accountant will help by setting up a bookkeeping system for you, auditing your books, and calculating your taxes and making out your returns. The bulk of the effort, though, will depend on you and your vigilance. One of the major reasons new businesses fail is inadequate financial management.

Proper financial management starts with record keeping. There are numerous types of records you will have to keep. This may seem tedious, but once you have the systems in place you'll find they are not so difficult, as long as you do your record keeping regularly. The government insists you keep accurate records, which provide the information for calculating your taxes. However, don't think that you keep records just to satisfy the government. These same records are among your most valuable management tools. Some of the records, for example, your daily journals and your profit and loss statements, give you a history of your business. They are your scorecard, so to speak. Other records, such as the budgets you prepare and your records of expenses, help you set your prices so your services make money. They also help you establish your goals by giving you an insight into where you are going. Your records help you create order out of chaos. They give you the facts you need to make sound business decisions. Your analysis of those facts will help you make realistic, logical choices on where to take your salon.

You do not have to become a bookkeeper or an accountant. You can hire them to do the actual work. But you will have to learn some basic bookkeeping and accounting terms and practices, just so you are able to understand what the numbers show.

There is a difference between bookkeeping and accounting. Bookkeeping refers to the mechanical and repetitive process of recording data. Accounting refers to the analysis and use of that data to provide detailed financial statements that furnish a basis for decision making. Your accountant can help you set up a system that works for you. The system you adopt should follow Generally Accepted Accounting Principles (GAAP), a series of standard procedures established by the accounting profession that is, in effect, the common language of accounting. If you have a computer in your salon, a number of programs are available that can simplify your record keeping. Your accountant can advise which program may be most useful for your operation.

FUNDAMENTALS OF BOOKKEEPING AND ACCOUNTING

The different kinds of records you'll keep vary in their time span. Some, like the journals, are kept daily; others are kept weekly, monthly, or quarterly. They will all follow the fiscal period you determine, which is usually one year long. Generally, the fiscal year for a business starts on January 1 and ends on December 31, although you can choose other starting and finishing points.

Your records, the books you keep, will show you the relationship between your assets, liabilities, and capital (also known as owner's equity or net worth). That relationship at any one time indicates the health of your business. It is the basic premise behind double-entry bookkeeping. The equation that describes the relationship is stated:

Assets = Liabilities + Capital

Assets are anything you own. These include your cash on hand, money in the bank, money owed to you (also known as your accounts receivable), supplies, and inventory, as well as your furniture, fixtures, and equipment. Liabilities are anything you owe. These include debts, bank loans, money owed on equipment or supplies (also known as your accounts payable). Capital is the monetary investment you (and your partners, if any) have made in the business. Capital goes on this side of the equation because it can be considered as money you owe to yourself. Capital is also sometimes called net worth.

Both sides of the equation must always be in balance, i. e., they must be equal. If you know two of the terms, you can find the third. Any transaction that occurs will change two of the terms of the equation to maintain that balance. For example, suppose your salon has assets of $10,000 and liabilities of $7,000. Your capital, then, is $3,000.

$10,000 = $7,000 + $3,000

Let's say you borrow $2,000 from the bank. Your assets increase to $12,000 with the added cash. However, your liabilities also increase to $9,000. Your capital remains at $3,000 and the equation is still in balance.

$12,000 = $9,000 + $3,000

But suppose, instead of borrowing the money, you invested another $2,000 of your own money. Your assets still increase to $12,000, but your liabilities remain $7,000 and your owner's equity increases to $5,000.

$$\$12,000 = \$7,000 + \$5,000$$

If you purchase a new piece of equipment, giving the manufacturer a promissory note, your assets increase by the amount of the value of the piece of equipment and your liabilities increase by the amount of the note. Let's assume you bought a new facial chair for $500 on credit. Your assets increase to $12,500, your liabilities increase to $7,500 and your capital stays at $5,000. If you paid cash, however, you still make two changes in the equation, but they both stay on the asset side. You increase your equipment account by $500 but decrease your cash account by the same amount. Your assets remain at $12,000, your liabilities at $7,000, and your capital at $5,000.

If your liabilities are greater than your assets, your owner's equity will be a negative number. Your business has no net worth and will not be in a healthy condition. You will either have to reduce your liabilities or increase your investment in the business to make your owner's equity positive. Although many businesses continue to operate with a deficit, this is definitely not a good practice.

The Daily Journal

Record keeping starts with your daily journal, a book in which you record the transactions of the day. You should make a written record of every transaction that occurs in your salon when it takes place, whether it involves cash coming in, credit given, or merchandise or cash going out. Each technician should write out a sales ticket for each customer, recording the customer's name, what service was received, and how much was paid. If the client purchases products for home use, record those on a separate ticket. (Your bookkeeping will be easier if you separate services from retail merchandise sales.)

By the same token, make a memo or receipt form for every transaction in which cash leaves the premises. These might include petty cash withdrawals, refunds, or cash purchases for incidental items, such as supplies for the salon's coffee pot, donations to a door-to-door solicitor, or cash reimbursement to an esthetician for tips charged to a credit card. Whenever possible, however, pay for purchases by business check. If you pay cash for anything, get a receipt.

At the close of the business day, transfer the data from the sales tickets and receipts into the journal in chronological order. Each entry in your journal should contain the date, a description of the transaction, and the amount that changed hands. Add up and record the income for the day, both cash and credit sales, then add up all monies that went out. Subtract the outgoing money from the income, and add the amount in the till at the start of the day. Then count the actual cash and credit vouchers on hand. The two amounts should be the same. If they are not, recheck the receipts. You should make every effort to account for shortages or overages.

The journal helps you keep accurate track of income and day-to-day expenses as they occur. The data you record here becomes the basis for your ledger as well as your balance sheet and other financial statements. In addition to providing financial data, the journal will serve as the salon's primary historical diary. It will give you a picture of which services are selling and which are not, the volume of each type of service, the activity of each cosmetologist, and the overall level of your business. It will also help you track your operating expenses. These data will let you forecast your future business and give you a basis for making sound operating decisions.

The Ledger

The ledger, also known as the general ledger, is your book of accounts, into which you enter information generated from the transactions recorded in your daily journal. It is the way you organize the data so you can use them most effectively. You establish an account—a separate reporting unit—for each asset, liability, income item, expense item, and owner's equity in the ledger. Each transaction is posted twice, once in a credit account and once in a debit account. Each account is entered in a T-shaped format; credits are placed on the right side; debits on the left side. The sum total of all the accounts—total debits equal total credits—must balance, although any individual account will not necessarily balance out. For each transaction, the dollar amount must be credited to one account and debited to another. You debit an account when you increase an asset or decrease a liability or owner's equity. Conversely, you credit an account when you decrease an asset or increase a liability or owner's equity. This format is the basis for the double-entry bookkeeping system, which is the most commonly used system, and allows for easy analysis of the information. The ledger shows you how the accounts change.

For example, suppose you purchased a magnifying lamp for your skin care treatment room. It cost $250 and you paid cash. Your cash on hand before the transaction was $5,000 and you had equipment valued at $4,000. You have decreased an asset, cash, by $250. You have increased a different asset, equipment, by $250. So, you credit your cash account and debit your equipment account by that amount. Your ledger accounts would be entered:

Cash		Equipment	
4750	250		250
		4000	

Now suppose, instead, you had acquired the lamp on credit. The same principles apply. You still debit your equipment account, but now you credit your accounts payable account because you have increased a liability. Your ledger accounts would now be entered:

Equipment		Accounts Payable	
250			250

A week later you pay off the promissory note for the lamp. You have decreased an asset, cash, by $250, and you have decreased a liability, accounts payable, by $250. Remember, a decrease in assets is a credit. A decrease in liabilities is a debit. Your ledger accounts are then entered:

Cash		Accounts Payable	
	250	250	

Note that in each case, the requirements of the standard book-keeping equation are met. Each transaction has had two effects and the debits and credits balance.

Unlike your daily journal, it is normally not necessary for you or your bookkeeper to make entries into the ledger every day. However, you should enter the data on a regular basis as often as is necessary to keep your books up-to-date. Making ledger entries weekly is usually sufficient.

The Balance Sheet

You, or your accountant, use the data from your daily journals and ledgers to create financial statements that let you analyze the health of your business. One of the most important of these statements is the balance sheet. This is a summary statement that lists your assets, liabilities, and owner's equity, and shows the financial condition of your salon as of a specific date. It follows the fundamental bookkeeping equation, with assets listed on the left and liabilities and owner's equity listed on the right, and both sides must be equal.

According to Generally Accepted Accounting Principles, assets are listed on the left side of the balance sheet in order of decreasing liquidity or their ready convertibility into cash. Liabilities are listed on the right side in order of the dates the debts come due. Owner's equity is also listed on the right side.

Current assets are listed first. These include cash, accounts receivable, inventory and prepaid expenses. Accounts receivable and inventory represent your highly liquid assets that can be bought, sold, and be converted back to cash within one normal operating cycle of your salon, typically within one year. Prepaid expenses include items such as rents paid in advance or payments for insurance policies. These are not liquid and can't be converted into cash, but are considered as current assets nonetheless.

Investments are listed next. These might include CDs, stocks, or other instruments into which you've put money. These are less liquid than current assets, but can still be converted into cash fairly easily.

Next in the assets column of the balance sheet come property, plant, and equipment. These are fixed, tangible assets that you own and were acquired for use in the normal operation of your salon and not for investment or for resale. Property refers to land and building sites; plant refers to buildings, facilities, and fixtures; equipment refers to the machinery and furniture you utilize to conduct your business. The dollar amount entered on the balance sheet for these is the acquisition cost (what you paid for them) adjusted for depreciation. Land, unlike plant and equipment, does not depreciate.

Finally, list intangible assets. These include items such as goodwill and customer records that you purchased. If you have trademarks, royalties, or patents, they are encompassed in this category. These items have almost no immediate cash value or liquidity, yet they are valuable resources that you own, so they must be accounted for. They are usually amortized over twenty to forty years.

On the liabilities, or right, side of the balance sheet, list current liabilities first. These include accounts payable, notes payable, wages payable, interest, and income taxes. Current liabilities are those debts incurred during the normal course of business and that must be paid in your normal operating cycle or within one year. These liabilities are normally paid from your existing current assets.

Next, list long-term liabilities. These include items such as bonds, loans payable over a period of years, and mortgages. In short, they cover your debts that will not come due within one year.

Your owner's equity is also entered on the right side of the balance sheet. Following the standard bookkeeping equation, when you add all the figures, the assets column should equal the total of the liabilities plus the owner's equity, or net worth of the salon.

From your balance sheet, you can determine your working capital. Subtract the current liabilities from the current assets. The excess is called working capital and determines your ability to finance your current operations. In short, it lets you know if you have enough cash to pay your bills. The relationship described by dividing your current assets by current liabilities is called the current ratio and is a measure of your liquidity and solvency. The larger the difference, the healthier your business. In a healthy business, that ratio should be about two to one or more.

You should generate a balance sheet at regular intervals, either monthly or quarterly as well as annually, depending on the particular needs of your salon. You can choose the fiscal period to cover. If you apply for financing, you will have to present your latest balance sheet and other records to the loan officer.

The Income Statement

The income statement is the other valuable financial statement. Like the balance sheet, the income statement describes the result of transactions during a specific time period, usually one month. Where the balance sheet is concerned with the relationship between assets, liabilities and net worth, however, the income statement is concerned with the relationship between revenues and expenses. Analyzing the balance sheet shows the profitability of your salon and net worth. Analyzing the income statement shows your cash flow.

The formula for the income statement starts with your net sales for the period—your gross sales of services and retail items minus returns, refunds, or other allowances. Subtract the cost of goods sold. For this category, you consider items you sell on the retail side of your salon as well as the materials you consume performing the services to determine the cost of the inventory you use. Net sales minus cost of goods sold gives you the gross profit, that is, your profit before you subtract operating expenses.

Next, subtract your operating and administrative expenses. These are all of the expenditures you make in the course of business except for inventory. They include items such as salaries, payroll taxes and benefit costs, rent, utilities, telephone, office supplies, advertising expenses, maintenance, insurance, postage, printing, legal and accounting fees, and depreciation. This gives you your operating profit, or your profit before nonoperating expenses or income.

Now, add any other income. This might include interest from savings or investments and rebates on materials. Then subtract other expenses, such as interest on loans. This gives you the net profit before tax, which is the figure you use to determine your income taxes. Then subtract the taxes. Your final number is your net profit after tax. This is what you get to keep and use, either to reinvest in the business, or as your personal income if you are a proprietor or partnership, or to distribute as dividends if you are a corporation. Remember the discussion on organization in Chapter 3. Proprietors and partners are not paid salaries; they share profits on which taxes have already been paid. In a corporation, owners can be paid salaries, on which they pay income taxes.

BUDGETS AND CASH MANAGEMENT

The information you get from the balance sheet and the income statement helps you manage your salon finances effectively. It lets you know exactly how your salon is doing and helps ensure survival. The single most important financial management step you can take is the management of cash, particularly your cash flow.

Cash flow is nothing more than the difference between income and disbursement and is as much a matter of timing as of dollar amounts. Cash almost always goes out before new cash comes in. You have to spend money, often before you generate any revenues. You must have enough cash available to finance your operations and acquire the things you need to make money. There may be a considerable lag between the time you spend the cash and get the payback. You need sufficient funds to overcome that time lag. To put it bluntly, if you run out of cash, you go out of business. This is a hard but incontrovertible fact of business life, especially for a small business with limited resources. It is necessary to balance inflow with outflow so you have cash available when you need it.

Don't be misled by your profit statement. Profits do not necessarily translate into cash. Profits are a bookkeeping concept, based on total assets, including inventory and accounts receivable. Cash is money in the bank. Profit is theory; cash is reality. You have to pay your bills in cash. You can't pay them with inventory or with money people owe you. Nor can you consider as cash all of the revenue that comes in. A certain portion of that revenue carries obligations, such as income tax payments, wages, and sales tax remissions. This doesn't mean you shouldn't be concerned with profit. Of course you should. Both cash and profit are essential to your business. Cash for survival; profit for good long-term business health.

Your cash flow situation is manageable, if you plan for it. Proper and timely planning will let you anticipate cash crunches and give you time to raise the funds you need. Your primary planning tool is your operating budget.

The operating budget is a projection of your expected revenues minus your expected expenses. It contains your estimates of how much cash will come into your salon, when it will come in, and where it will come from, as well as your estimates of how much your expenses will be and when they will be paid. It is your blueprint for cash flow.

You generate this budget from your forecasts of sales and other cash income and the expenses you can expect to face. The operating budget is similar to the capital budget you generated when you were planning the start-up of your salon. Unlike that budget, however, this budget covers a shorter time, usually a year, although it should list projected income and expenses on a monthly basis.

Since the budget is based on estimates and not on actual data, it will not be completely accurate, especially when you have just started your business. But as long as it has been carefully conceived, it will serve as a valuable planning guide. As you acquire actual sales and expense figures, you should revise your budget frequently. Make your estimates realistically and objectively and think through your assumptions thoroughly. It is better to underestimate your revenues and overestimate your expenses.

When you develop your budget, be careful not to overlook any operating expenses. Also consider how you are going to live during this period. You need food to eat and a place to sleep. Do you have a separate income to meet your daily personal needs, or will you have to draw funds out of the business? If so, factor those into the budget, too.

Budget for contingencies, as well. Set aside funds to cover emergencies such as repairs, maintenance, or unexpected replacement of equipment. For example, what will you do if your water heater breaks? Even if it is covered by insurance, you will have to replace the appliance immediately. You won't have time to wait for the insurance check. You can't always foresee what might go wrong, so you'd better have enough cash on hand to meet crises as they occur.

PRICE MANAGEMENT

The revenues coming into your salon depend on the number of customers you service and how much you charge them for the services. The prices you establish go a long way toward determining your success. If they're too low, you might lose money. If they're too high, you may lose customers. Setting prices is more an art than a science. There are a lot of factors involved, not all of them are financial. Your accountant will be able to help you establish your prices.

As a starting point, you must first determine what each service costs. Calculate both the direct costs and the indirect costs. First, list all of the services you offer. Determine the cost of supplies used to perform each service. This is the direct cost of the service. Take for example, a leg waxing. Assume it takes thirty minutes. The only supplies used are the wax and muslin strips, which cost fifty cents. It may seem like nit-picking to consider amounts this small, but they all add up. Even little expenses are important. In this case, your direct costs are fifty cents. In a service business such as a skin and body care salon, direct costs are generally low.

Your indirect costs, however, are much higher but no less real. These are harder to figure because you have to consider averages. The indirect costs are a function of your operating and administrative expenses, divided by the number of customers you expect to service in a given time period. This gives you an average cost per customer, which you add to the direct cost of the service.

For example, assume you have four hundred customers a month. Add up your expenses for the month, including rent, insurance, utilities, telephone, advertising, taxes, and accounting and legal services. Don't add the cost of materials. You've already considered that in the direct cost. Let's say your expenses for the month are $2,500. Now add in the cost of your employees. This includes salaries, your share of Social Security taxes withheld, and benefits. Don't forget to include your draw if you are taking any money from the salon. Assume your labor costs for the month are $2,500. Your total indirect labor and overhead costs are $5,000. Divide that by four hundred customers. Your total indirect cost per customer is $12.50. Add that to the direct cost to get your total cost of the service. In the case of the leg waxing, it is $0.50 plus $12.50 for a total of $13.00. So, it costs you $13.00 to sell one leg waxing. Other services will be more or less, depending on the cost of materials used.

This is your break-even price. If you set your price lower, you will lose money. If you set it higher, you will make money. How much higher you will set the price depends on the profit margin you are comfortable with, what similar services at competitive salons cost, and how much the clientele you've targeted are willing and able to pay. Also, you will want to set aside some of the income to finance future growth.

Don't assume that you will have to charge the same prices for your services that other salons in the area charge for theirs. You may be able to charge more if you are offering service quality and competence of which they are incapable. You also have to consider the image you want your salon to project. If you position your salon as an exclusive, high-quality, high-class operation, you can charge more. If you position your salon as a low-cost, volume operation, you will charge less.

EXPENSE MANAGEMENT

You can see from the hypothetical cost analysis that your four hundred customers must generate $5,000 plus the cost of your materials in sales, just so you'll break even for the month. There are only two ways you can change your indirect average cost per customer. Either you increase the number of customers or you reduce your expenses. It is very important that you keep tight control on your expenses as they can easily get out of hand and wreck your profitability.

Expenses, like the need for cash, are a fact of business life. The efficient management of expenses, like the management of your cash flow, can make or break your operation. Some expenses you can control; others you cannot. But you must be aware of all of the expenses you face and be prepared for them.

Your operating expenses are those items that are necessary for the direct conduct of your business. These include the supplies you use for the services you provide, the inventory of products you sell, and services you purchase, such as towel and uniform rentals. These expenses will vary with your customer flow. The more customers you get, the higher these will go, but not necessarily proportionately. You can also control these expenses to some extent. For example, you can lower your supply costs by shopping for the best deals and by keeping your inventory levels low.

Your labor costs are also operating expenses, but depend on the number of employees you have and your compensation levels. Salaries are the major expense, but there are other expenses connected with employees, as well. You also have to consider the costs of benefit packages, such as hospitalization, your share of Social Security taxes, and workers' compensation and unemployment insurance charges that may be levied by the state in which you do business. You might also factor in costs for sending key employees to training courses. These costs will vary with the number of employees you have.

You can control the labor costs by keeping that number low. Have only as many employees as you actually need to do the work, but have enough to do the work properly. You can cut your staff too thin. Use some part-time workers instead of all full-time employees. You might also have some employees perform more than one task. For example, your receptionist may double as your bookkeeper or may handle your retail sales. Of course, you will have to pay them accordingly, although paying one person more will still be lower than paying two people less.

Administrative, or overhead, expenses are necessary for the indirect conduct of your business. These include fixed expenses such as rent, utilities, telephone, insurance, license fees, trash removal, and water and sewer rent. These costs generally stay the same month to month and are not affected by the level of business you conduct. There are some variable administrative expenses, too. These include professional fees, advertising, printing, postage, interest payments on loans and notes, and payments on loan principals.

You can control some of these costs. Advertising costs, for example, will vary with the level of advertising you conduct and with the media you utilize. Except for telephone directory advertising, which you purchase on a yearly basis, you can schedule advertising to fit monthly cash availability. (This may not be the most effective way to advertise, but if you need to reduce expenses, it is a way to do it.) The fees you pay your accountant and lawyer will vary with the amount of work they do in a given month. Interest payments become lower as the principal is reduced, and you can lower monthly payments on interest and principal by renegotiating loan terms.

Then there are the unexpected expenses. Something breaks and needs to be repaired or replaced. Someone gets sick and you need to hire temporary help. One of your suppliers is offering a deal on equipment or supplies that it would be prudent to accept. You can't anticipate everything that will happen at any given moment in your business. But you can anticipate that something unexpected—and expensive—will happen. That something will be just as real an expense as any of the other expenses you face. Your only recourse is to have planned for contingencies and have funds set aside to meet them.

So manage your expenses wisely, and control them whenever you can. Expense management is every bit as important as cash flow management. Make decisions about your expenses as prudently as you make decisions about any other aspect of your business.

TAXATION

Taxes are another expense you will face. They are an inexorable fact of business life. They come from virtually every level of government and in many forms. The requirements for calculating your tax obligations vary widely from tax to tax, from state to state, and from community to community. The rules are complicated and change almost without warning. This is one area where it is mandatory to have professional help. Your accountant may, in fact, perform his or her most valuable service in the area of taxation.

There are many kinds of tax. At the federal level, there are income taxes, paid on profits in a manner determined by the organization of your business—sole proprietorship, partnership, S-corporation or C-corporation. There are also Social Security (FICA) taxes, paid equally by the employee and the employer. On the state level, there are state income taxes and sales and use taxes, which you must collect from your customers and pass on to the state sales tax agency. On the community level, there are an assortment of business, wage, occupation, and school taxes.

Your accountant will tell you which taxes apply to you, and will calculate your tax liability. The accounting controls he or she has set up for you and the care and accuracy with which you have kept your records will help make sure that you pay no more taxes than you owe.

Taxes are necessary. It is how we pay for the services we receive from the government. Federal and state government programs are funded through taxes. Police protection, fire protection, and schools are funded through local taxes. It is a duty to pay your tax obligations. It is not a duty to pay more than you owe, however. It's not unpatriotic to limit your taxes by taking advantage of deductions allowed by the tax laws. For example, travel to another city to take a course in business management or to attend a trade meeting is deductible. Books and materials you purchase to help you conduct your business are also deductible. But follow your accountant's advice and don't overdo the deductions.

Tax evasion, however, is illegal. It is a criminal offense, punishable by imprisonment and fines, to deliberately avoid paying your legitimate taxes. Failure to make tax payments when they are due, even if not done with criminal intent, will cause you problems. You will be liable for interest and fines on the unpaid taxes. Your business may be padlocked shut, and your property, business as well as personal, can be seized.

If you are in a cash crunch, you can sometimes defer payments to suppliers and to lending institutions if you approach them early and renegotiate terms. You cannot defer tax payments, so keep your tax obligations uppermost in mind when you make your cash flow projections. They are an integral part of your financial management package.

BANKRUPTCY

Bankruptcy. It's a fearful term, but it can happen when you don't manage your finances properly. Remember the cash flow credo—out of cash; out of luck. However, bankruptcy proceedings can also be a management tool that will help your business get out of financial trouble and buy you time to solve your problems. It does not necessarily put you out of business.

Before you consider bankruptcy proceedings, however, you should contact your creditors and inform them of your payment problems. Be honest with them, treat them all equally, and let them know about the problems as early as possible. Don't wait until the last minute. Chances are they will renegotiate terms, giving you longer to pay or remitting some charges. It is in their best interests to renegotiate, since they will probably recover more money than if you declared bankruptcy.

Get professional help. Work with your attorney and your accountant to develop a workable plan for repayment and present that plan to the creditors. Once you have an agreement, keep to the terms. If this doesn't work, your alternative is to declare bankruptcy.

Bankruptcy is a court supervised procedure that works to protect both sides as much as possible and arrange mutually acceptable solutions. It can be voluntary (you initiate proceedings) or involuntary (your creditors force it upon you). Bankruptcy proceedings are covered by the federal Bankruptcy Act and supersede any state laws. The bankruptcy court protects you from your creditors. Once proceedings have begun, creditors cannot take any independent collection measures. The court will discharge your debts as equitably as possible, giving you an opportunity to start over. The only debts that cannot be discharged by bankruptcy are taxes and such items as alimony payments.

The federal Bankruptcy Act specifies a number of types of bankruptcy. Chapter 7 bankruptcy is the most common type and involves liquidation of assets. This is the form you would use when your finances are totally out of control and you have no hope of recovering. Proceedings under this chapter can be voluntary or involuntary. Under Chapter 7, the court appoints a trustee who oversees the sale of your assets and distributes the money among the creditors. Whatever debts remain after the money is distributed are discharged. It dismantles and shuts down the business. If you are a sole proprietor or a partnership, both your business assets and your personal property can be sold.

You can retain some of your property rights, however. Federal and state laws allow some exemptions. You can choose either the federal exemptions or those allowed by the state in which you reside. For example, under the federal statutes, you can keep $7,500 equity in your house and $1,200 equity in your car. You also keep your rights to Social Security and pension benefits. Once the proceedings are closed and remaining debts are discharged, you are free to start another business, but you cannot file for bankruptcy under Chapter 7 for a period of six years.

An alternative to Chapter 7 is to file for bankruptcy under Chapter 11. Proceedings under this chapter may be initiated voluntarily or involuntarily. Unlike Chapter 7, which liquidates the business and sells the assets, Chapter 11 gives you relief from your creditors while you reorganize the business. The court forms a committee of creditors, which helps you devise a plan for repayment of your debts. Once you file under Chapter 11, you have 120 days to develop a plan for reorganization. After that time, the creditors can force a plan on you. Once the plan is confirmed by the court, all parties are bound by its provisions. If the plan doesn't work and you keep losing money, the court can convert the Chapter 11 proceedings into a Chapter 7 bankruptcy. The Chapter 11 bankruptcy lets you keep the business going.

If you are a sole proprietor, you have another choice. You can file for bankruptcy under Chapter 13, which was developed for individuals. This form is strictly voluntary. Your creditors cannot force you into it. Under a court-appointed trustee's supervision, you develop a plan to adjust your debts and repay your creditors. Once the court approves the plan, your creditors can't harass you. The court will grant you this protection for three years, but may extend it to five years. While you are under the court's protection, your creditors can't force you to liquidate the business.

Bankruptcy is not a step to be taken lightly, but you should not fear it. It can help you out of financial trouble and give you extra time to get your business in order. Bankruptcy laws are complicated, however, so it is vital that you have the help of your lawyer and accountant to lead you through the pitfalls and problems. Don't be afraid to ask them for help. Seek their advice and follow their recommendations.

Your best choice, though, is to follow good financial management practices. Watch your cash flow and monitor your expenses. If you take care not to get into financial trouble, you won't have to worry about bankruptcy.

SUMMARY

For your salon to be profitable, you must manage it according to sound financial practices. This takes painstaking record keeping. While your accountant and bookkeeper will do much of this work, you must understand the principles so you can analyze the records and evaluate where you are profitable and where you are not. In short, these records tell you how healthy your business is.

There are a number of records you will have to keep. Your daily journal keeps track of all transactions that occur in your salon each day, whether it involves cash coming in or going out, the services performed, and the merchandise sold or returned. Each of your employees should keep meticulous records. Your ledger organizes the data you generate, so you can use the information.

The data from both the ledger and the daily journal forms the basis for the information that goes into your balance sheet, a summary statement that shows your financial condition at any given point and shows you the relationship between your assets, liabilities, and net worth. The income statement, on the other hand gives you the results of all transactions and shows you the relationship between revenues and expenses.

Cash flow, the difference in dollars between what comes into the salon and what goes out, is an important consideration in financial management. You must make sure you have adequate amounts of cash on hand to run your business properly. If you don't have enough cash, you will go out of business.

You can manage your cash flow situation if you plan for it. The tool for doing this is your budget. The budget projects your estimates for both income and expenses. When you prepare your budget, don't forget to allow for the unexpected.

It is also necessary to manage your expenses. You can enhance your cash flow and profitability by keeping your expenses as low as possible. This takes a lot of care. It is very easy to waste resources.

But it is vital that you take the effort in this area. Don't forget to consider taxes. There are many taxes you will face in business, and it is necessary to pay them. Failure to do so can lead to catastrophic consequences.

When you fail to manage your cash flow and your expenses properly, you can go bankrupt. But there are different forms of bankruptcy. Choosing the proper course of action can help you get out of financial trouble and bring your business back on course. To do this, however, you will need the help and advice of your accountant and your attorney.

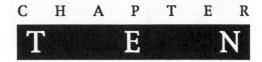

One of the most difficult tasks you'll face as a salon owner or manager is hiring a competent staff. It is also one of the most important jobs you'll have. Almost more than any other factor, the staff you assemble can make or break your salon. Your employees are the people who interface with your customers and who perform the services the customers pay for. How well they perform those services, their attitudes and demeanor, will determine whether or not those customers will come back.

How well your employees perform and how appropriately they behave is a direct result of your competence as a personnel manager. If you hire the right people, and train and motivate them properly, they will respond and your business will prosper. If you hire the wrong people, don't train or motivate them, your business will suffer.

As personnel administrator, your objective is to assemble a team that will work together to make the salon profitable. Ideally, the staff members should complement each other, that is, each bring a skill or an attitude to the job that the others can learn and profit from. Your staff should develop a synergy so that the whole should be greater than the sum of the parts. And the group should be able to work well together. How well they do that depends, in a large part, on the attitudes and skills you bring to the salon. If you don't care about your business, they certainly won't. You set the tone for your salon. Your employees will follow your lead.

Your employees have the right to expect you to be fair, honest, consistent, and responsive to their concerns. In turn, you have the right to expect loyalty, honesty, and responsibility from them. This requires an atmosphere of trust, which comes from maintaining open lines of two-way communication. It is very easy for you, as the owner or manager, to get so involved in other aspects of the business that you forget the needs of your employees. It is equally easy for you to fall into the trap of thinking you always know what's best for your business. Don't let your ego get in the way of your relationship with your staff. Make them an integral part of your business, and let them know that each and every one is important to you. Listen to them. Seek out their suggestions and ideas, act on those that have merit, and share the rewards.

But remember, also, that it is necessary for you to keep some distance from your employees. Anyone you hire you may have to fire, so it is important that you not be friends with staff members. You can and should be friendly with all of them, however. No matter how much you may not like this idea, you must always be aware that you are the boss. The ultimate responsibility for the success of your salon rests with you, not with your employees.

SALON POSITIONS

Depending on the skin and body care services you offer and the size of your salon, you will need to fill a number of positions. Each position performs a certain function in the salon. Some may be more skilled than others, but all are important to the smooth and efficient function of the business. Also, consider what functions you and your partners (if any) will perform. Will you be strictly an administrator and manager? Will you be an absentee owner? Or will you also perform skin care or other functions? For staffing purposes, consider yourself and your partners as employees if you are going to be physically present in the salon.

Don't overstaff. Hire only the help you need to get the job done. You can hire more people as your business grows and you need them. It is better for your employees to be busy, even slightly overworked, than it is to have them spending a lot of idle time. They will be happier, since they'll have the potential to earn more money, and

CHECKLIST 10-1
SALON POSITIONS

Position	Primary Duties
Receptionist	Book appointments
	Collect payment for services
	Maintain reception area
Esthetician	Perform facials and body care services
Massage Therapist	Perform body massages
Electrologist	Perform electrolysis services
Makeup Stylist	Apply makeup
	Give consultation services
	Sell cosmetics
Manicurist	Perform manicures
	Perform pedicures
Retail Sales Clerk	Sell products
Manager	Coordinate and run salon functions

you'll be happier because your bottom line will be better. Not all your employees need to work full-time. You can hire part-time employees to fill certain positions, either for peak periods of activity, such as on weekends or holidays, or to perform currently under-utilized services. Also remember that some of your employees may be able to fill more than one position. For example, your receptionist might also double as your retail sales clerk. Utilize your staff's abilities as fully as you can.

Write a comprehensive job description for each position. This document should describe fully the duties and responsibilities of the position. The written job description defines the function and sets the parameters for filling it, lets the employee know what he or she is expected to do, and can help resolve disputes or misunderstandings over work assignments. Give the employee a copy before he or she accepts the job. Make sure he or she understands it and agrees with it. You can revise the document as the position evolves, but you may have to negotiate changes with employees you've already hired in the position.

The positions you might need to fill can include one or more of each of the following:

Receptionist. Although not a "skill" position, like an esthetician, the receptionist plays a key role in the salon. He or she is the first contact with the customers and functions as the salon's "traffic cop," to keep people and services moving smoothly. The receptionist books appointments, collects payments for services, maintains the reception area, and sees to the needs of clients while they are waiting. He or she may also maintain the customer data base and sell retail products, among many other activities.

The receptionist does not need a license but should be thoroughly trained in the services the salon offers and in the scheduling time requirements of each of the estheticians and other technicians. He or she should also be familiar with the products offered for retail sale and be able to answer questions about their use. More than most other staff members, the receptionist needs to be a people person. He or she needs an outgoing personality and must enjoy dealing with the public.

Esthetician. The esthetician performs facials, waxing, and body care services. This is a highly skilled specialty and requires an esthetician license. With additional training in the specialty, one who holds a cosmetology license may also perform the services. Although the esthetician can also perform manicuring and other services if he or she has a cosmetology license, the field is so specialized that he or she should limit practice to esthetics services.

Massage Therapist. If your salon offers such services, you might want to employ a massage therapist. Although the esthetician can perform most massage services, the function requires a high level of skill and training. The esthetician will require additional training to perform these services competently. In some states, the practitioner must hold a massage therapist license.

Electrologist. The electrologist performs electrolysis services and is a specialist in the field. He or she must have specific training and, in most states, must hold an electrologist license. Like the esthetician or massage therapist, this position also requires a very high level of skill, training, and expertise.

Makeup Stylist. The makeup stylist applies and sells cosmetics. This is also a salon specialty that requires skill and training, though not at the same high skill level of other salon services. Although the makeup stylist may not be required to hold a license in some states, others may require that he or she hold a cosmetology license. He or she must be competent and have specific training in makeup application services. An esthetician may be able to fill this position in addition to his or her other duties.

Manicurist. The manicurist performs the full range of manicure and pedicure services in the salon. This is a skill position and requires either a manicurist or cosmetologist license. Although the manicurist is an important part of the staff, the position does not require as high a skill level as the estheticians. The manicurist should be familiar with current practices and should be capable of performing advanced techniques, such as nail tipping and nail painting.

Retail Sales Clerk. The sales clerk sells the retail products you offer in the salon and may also be responsible for ordering and stocking the products. The clerk also maintains the retail sales area. Unless your salon is heavily involved in retail sales, you will probably not need a full-time sales clerk. This function may be handled by the receptionist or another designated employee. In some salons, each employee is responsible for selling products to his or her clients.

Manager. The manager coordinates and runs all of the functions of the salon and is ultimately responsible for the efficiency and profitability of the business. Unless either you or a partner are managing the salon, you will have to hire a manager. In most states, this person must hold a salon manager's license and will have had specific training in salon management practices. If you are the salon owner, you do not need a manager's license, nor are you required to have any specialized training in management. This is a pity, because if you do not have training and expertise in management practices, your salon may not survive.

The manager may also work as an esthetician or perform other functions. You may also designate another employee to act as manager in your absence.

INDEPENDENT CONTRACTORS

In addition to your employees, you may also hire a number of independent contractors. These are people who perform services for your business, but who are not employed by you. They operate their own businesses and do not receive a salary or benefits from you. This category includes such people as your lawyer, accountant, bookkeeper, or cleaning service. These various functions have been discussed in other chapters.

It is important to understand the distinction between an independent contractor and an employee. As an employer, you are responsible for withholding certain taxes, such as Social Security taxes and federal, state, and local income taxes, from your employees, and must pay other taxes, such as unemployment insurance and matching Social Security taxes. In an effort to circumvent this responsibility, some salon owners have rented space to persons in exchange for a portion of the income they generate. They have then classified these people as independent contractors and have not withheld taxes, leaving payment up to the individual.

If you are considering such a practice, be very careful. First, in some states, the practice may be illegal under the state cosmetology regulations. Second, the IRS may consider those people as employees anyway, and hold you liable for back taxes, interest, and severe penalties. The difference between an employee and an independent contractor depends largely on the amount of control you exercise. If you determine such things as working hours and how the work will be done, or if you supply the space or the equipment, the IRS will most likely consider that person an employee. If you have any questions about the classification of people in your salon, consult your lawyer or accountant. You can also find information in IRS Publication 539, *Employment Taxes*, which discusses the relationship between employee and employer.

TAX INFORMATION FOR EMPLOYERS

As an employer, you are responsible for collecting and paying several different taxes. Some of these are your responsibility, others are the responsibility of the employees, but you must withhold the money from their pay and send it to the government. You must also keep meticulous records of the amounts withheld and submitted. Work closely with your accountant to establish the amounts to withhold and to set up a schedule for meeting federal, state, and local tax payments. Read IRS Circular E, *Employer's Tax Guide*, and IRS Publication 583,

Taxpayers Starting a Business, for information on your federal tax requirements. Call your state revenue department for information on your state tax responsibilities, and check with your community for local tax requirements.

Employee Records

The IRS requires that you keep accurate records of all employee transactions. You must first file Form SS-4 with the IRS to obtain your Employer Identification Number (EIN), which you must put on all of the federal and state tax returns you submit. If you are a sole proprietorship, you may use your Social Security number as your taxpayer identification number, instead of the EIN. Then you must get each employee's Social Security number. Make sure you verify the accuracy of that number by reading it directly from the employee's Social Security card.

Each employee must fill out IRS Form W-4, *Employee's Withholding Allowance Certificate,* in which he or she claims withholding exemptions. In addition, each employee must fill out Form I-9, Employment Eligibility Verification Form, which is available from the Immigration and Naturalization Service, to verify that he or she is either a citizen or legal alien and can legally work in this country. The employee must complete this form within three days of being hired.

You must keep files on employees for a minimum of four years, preferably longer. The information you must keep includes employee name and address, Social Security number, the position filled, and the dates of employment. You also need to keep all W-4 and I-9 forms, as well as all salary information. This includes dates and amounts of payments for wages and benefits, such as vacation and sick pay, or contributions to pension plans or medical and life insurance plans. It also includes tips, which are reported to the IRS on Form 8027, *Employer's Information Return of Tip Income.*

It is also necessary to keep records on tax payments you make. Keep your cancelled checks and all copies of Form 8109, *Federal Tax Deposit Coupon,* and Form 941, *Quarterly Return of Withheld Income Tax and Social Security Taxes.* Also keep copies of Form 940, Federal Unemployment Tax returns and any state return forms you utilize. Your accountant and lawyer can advise you of federal, state, and local record keeping requirements.

Employee Tax Liabilities

Employees are liable for federal, state, and local income taxes and for Social Security taxes. As the employer, you must withhold these taxes from their pay and make periodic payments to the Internal Revenue Service. For most small businesses, these payments are made quarterly, although larger firms may be required to make payments more often. Remember too, that tips are taxable. Your employees must report the amount of tips they receive to you. In turn, you must report that to the IRS on Form 8027. You will also have to withhold applicable state and local income and occupation taxes.

In-kind services may also be taxable. For example, if your employees receive free facials or manicures, the IRS considers those to be part of the employees' compensation. Taxes should be paid on the fair value of those services.

Employer Tax Liabilities

Your tax liabilities, as an employer, include the matching portion of the Social Security taxes. The employee pays half, which you withhold from his or her salary, and you pay half. You are also responsible for paying federal and state unemployment taxes. These tax revenues finance programs to provide compensatory payments to employees who are laid off or fired from their jobs for lack of work. Employees who are fired for cause, that is, for insubordination or misconduct, are not eligible for unemployment compensation.

You must also pay a self-employment tax, which is the Social Security tax for self-employed people. The rate is approximately the same as the rate at which you withhold Social Security taxes for your employees, plus your matching contribution. For more information, see IRS Publication 533, *Self-Employment Tax.*

You will also pay the Federal Unemployment (FUTA) tax, which funds unemployment insurance programs. This tax is separate from Social Security taxes and is paid only by employers. It is not withheld from employees' pay.

Another payment you will have to make, although not strictly speaking a tax, is for workers' compensation insurance. All states require employers to carry such insurance, which pays medical expenses and disability benefits to workers who are injured while on the job. Requirements vary from state to state, so contact your state labor department for information.

The taxes discussed in this section deal only with those applicable to employment practices. You are responsible for a host of other taxes, which are discussed in other chapters. The government has set strict guidelines for compliance with the tax laws, and penalties for noncompliance are severe. Mistakes are costly, so work closely with your accountant to avoid problems.

FINDING AND HIRING EMPLOYEES

You know which positions you need to fill to assemble your team. Now, you have to find the people to fill them. This is much more difficult than it seems. Good employees are a scarce commodity and hard to find. They are even harder to keep.

You know the attributes you want in your employees. They have to be competent, of course, and possess the skill and experience to perform the services well and quickly. But competence is not enough. They also have to be able to satisfy and work with their clients. You need people with a positive attitude who enjoy working with people and who are willing to do what's necessary to advance. They should be ambitious, and look to the future, without being ruthless. They should be assertive without being aggressive. And they should be presentable, that is, clean in body and in manner. Social skills are just as important as performance skills.

Now consider why anyone would want to work for you. What do you offer that makes your salon a more inviting place to work than the competition? And make no mistake. You will be competing with other salons for the best employees. You have to sell your salon to the prospective employee just as much as he or she has to sell his or her abilities to you.

Salon Information Package

As your first step, develop an information package that details the benefits of working at your salon. This will accomplish two things. First, it will make you think about the things you have to offer; second, it will give you a tool to use in your recruiting efforts. The package should include photographs of your salon, preferably showing people working, that show it as bright, attractive, and well-designed. Include a description and history of your salon. Talk about your philosophy of doing business, include the mission statement from your business plan, and list the advantages of working for you, such as training, and opportunities for advancement. Add any benefits you offer, such as bonuses, vacations, paid holidays, and health insurance.

Add job descriptions of all of the positions, outlining their duties and responsibilities. Also include a list of all the services you offer in the salon, along with prices. Finally, enclose an application form.

This salon information package is your first representative. It will create an impression in the minds of prospective employees. Whether that impression will be favorable or unfavorable depends on the care and attention you take to develop the package. Spend the money it takes to do the job right. After all, you spend money on advertising to attract clients. Why shouldn't you spend some money to attract employees?

Prospect Sources

Now, where do you find prospects? There are a number of sources. Ideally, of course, you'd like to hire experienced people with followings. To reach these people, you can advertise in the classified want-ad sections of local newspapers. Want ads can be effective, but you should be specific about the job requirements. Direct the advertisement to the people you are trying to attract. Give some hint about your salon, but not too much. You are trying to arouse interest. So, for example, your ad might read:

> Experienced esthetician with following wanted for full-time position in busy, modern center-city skin care salon. Excellent working conditions and benefit package for the right person. Call 555-1234 to arrange for interview and audition.

The ad states your requirements—an experienced esthetician with a following—it gives some idea of the job, characterizes your salon, and offers an inducement to respond. And it invites a response. If you don't want prospects to call you directly, most newspapers offer a blind box response mechanism, where prospects write to a specific box number. The newspaper then forwards the responses to you.

If you need more than one stylist, say so in the ad. But, limit each ad to one kind of position. If you need, for example, an esthetician and a manicurist, run two separate ads. Another key to a successful want ad is frequency. You have to run the ad enough times for it to be effective. You should run the ad on a daily basis for at least one week, in as many relevant media as you can find. If your community or its surroundings has more than one daily newspaper, advertise in all of them. Classified ads are relatively inexpensive, and once the positions are filled, you can stop advertising. But keep the resumes and applications of all the qualified people who responded on file. They can be a source for future hiring when other positions open.

Employment agencies and job placement services are another source for finding experienced salon employees. Employers register with the agency or service and provide them with a list of positions and qualifications. Job seekers register with these agencies and provide a list of their abilities and requirements. In addition the agencies advertise positions available and engage in other recruiting efforts. The agency or service then matches applicants with employers and arranges for interviews.

The advantage of these services is that they organize and manage the recruiting efforts and provide the initial screening of candidates, so you only see the people that meet your requirements. The disadvantages are cost and a lack of exclusivity. Any agency may be soliciting candidates for more than one salon. Some agencies charge fees based on salary amounts. The employer pays a fee and so does the successful job applicant. Other services charge the employer a registration fee, which may be several hundred dollars each year but covers an unlimited number of applicant searches. And you pay no additional fees if you hire someone they recommend.

You may also solicit employees at other salons. If you know of a good esthetician or other employee who works at another salon, there is nothing illegal or unethical about asking them to come and work for you. You can do this yourself or through an intermediary, such as one of your customers or another employee, or you can hire a professional recruiter to handle the negotiations. The advantage of this approach is that you can target specific individuals that you know are good workers. The disadvantage is that other salon owners or recruiters may also be soliciting your employees.

Use your own employees as recruiters. They may have friends and acquaintances in the business. Offer incentives to your staff members to suggest prospective employees. These can take the form of monetary payments for each person they recruit, once you've hired the person and he or she has worked for a specific period of time.

Beauty schools usually offer job placement services for both new and past graduates. Establish relationships with the beauty schools in your area. Participate in their career days and other programs. Give them a supply of your salon information kits. Schools are often a good source for finding experienced help.

Don't limit your recruiting practices to finding only experienced employees. You may find it profitable and rewarding to hire new beauty school graduates and train them. As long as they have the talent and the desire to do well and to advance in their trade, and are willing to start at the bottom, you have the opportunity to develop a productive, long-term employee.

As long as you are in business, you will never stop recruiting. Even when you are fully staffed, continue to accept applications and keep them on file. You never know when you'll have to hire someone new, either because an employee has quit or because your business has grown enough to let you expand your services. That applicant file will become a primary source for new hires.

Interviews and Auditions

Once you have identified potential employees, it is necessary to assess their work and social skills and determine which of them you want to hire. You do this through interviews and auditions. These are a vital part of the hiring process. Be careful how you conduct your interviews. There are many legal considerations involved. You must be aware of privacy and discrimination matters, and how they can affect your hiring decisions.

Every applicant should provide a resume, with references, and should fill out a job application form. This form is a legal document that you should keep on file whether or not you hire the person. It should ask only for information that is directly related to the prospect's ability to perform the job. It should promise nothing. The application becomes a permanent part of the employee's records and anything contained in the form could come back to haunt you. When you develop your application form, have your attorney review it before you have it printed. Then, have him or her periodically rereview the document to make sure it continues to follow current legal requirements.

Before setting up the interview, examine the applicant's resume and application. Look for work history and education, as they apply to the job for which he or she is applying. Check all of the applicant's references. Then, when you are satisfied that he or she may be suitable for your salon, conduct the interview.

The interview is a two-way process. It is a face-to-face opportunity to learn about the abilities and interests of the applicant, and is his or her opportunity to learn about you and your salon. Both of you should benefit from the experience. Pay attention not only to what the applicant says, but also to what he or she does. Was the applicant on time for the appointment? Was he or she neatly dressed and groomed? What kind of demeanor did the applicant show? These are all indications of work habits and attitudes.

Let the applicant do most of the talking. Ask specific questions, but make sure they have a bearing on job performance. If there are inconsistencies on the resume and application, make sure you ask about these. You may ask about education, status of licenses, and work experience. You may not ask about such personal matters as marital status, age, religion, or health, unless these questions have a demonstrable bearing on the person's ability to do the job.

Answer applicant's questions truthfully and fully, but be careful. When you are discussing the salon, don't promise anything you can't deliver. For example, don't talk about tenure or annual raises. Anything you promise during the interview or list on the application form could be ruled an implied contract, and you could be held to its terms.

At the end of the interview, if you are interested in the applicant, you can schedule the audition. This tests the applicant's skills and can show you how well he or she actually performs the work. It can also indicate the applicant's work habits and ability to work with customers. Observe the applicant carefully during the audition. This phase of the hiring process is just as important as the interview.

The Hiring Offer

Once you have finished the interviews and auditions, you're ready to make the hiring decision. Choose the applicant you want to hire, then extend the job offer. This is the time to negotiate salary and benefits with the prospective employee. Although these terms are negotiable, and you can be flexible, they should not vary widely from guidelines you have established as part of your salon policies.

When you consider which applicant to hire, keep antidiscrimination laws in mind. The law says you may not discriminate against any applicant because of race, sex, national origin, age, or religion in your hiring, promotion, training, or compensation practices. Unintentional discrimination is just as illegal as intentional discrimination.

Make sure all the terms of employment are clear—duties, work hours, salary, benefits, and salon policies. If the applicant accepts, you have a new employee, and a new set of responsibilities. To protect yourself, and the employee, keep a written record of all agreements you've made in his or her file. Give the employee a copy of your salon's Employee Handbook. Make sure he or she reads and understands it, and have him or her sign a statement to that effect.

Establish a reasonable probationary period (three to six months) during which you can assess the employee's work and attitudes, and make sure the employee realizes that he or she is on probation. At the end of the period, give the successful employee a reward, such as a pay increase. You have much more freedom to terminate an employee who isn't working out during the probationary period than you do afterwards.

The positive attitudes and motivation of your employees starts from their first day of employment. Make sure you introduce your new hire to other staff members. Assign a mentor, an experienced employee, to help the new employee adjust to his or her new surroundings. Make the new employee feel like part of the team right from the beginning.

KEEPING EMPLOYEES

Hiring good employees is difficult; keeping them can be even harder. Employees are always free to leave. It's up to you to create a working environment that will make them want to stay. That environment starts with your attitudes toward fairness, honesty, and opportunity. It continues with your encouragement and motivation. And it depends on your consistency and responsiveness to the legitimate concerns of the employees.

Fairness means managing your staff in an evenhanded manner. It means having established practices in your salon and enforcing those practices equally among all staff members. Treat everyone the same. Don't play favorites. This is why you should be careful about hiring friends or relatives. No matter how hard you may try to be fair, any promotions or perks you give to them will be perceived, whether rightly or wrongly, as giving them an unfair advantage. A good boss is friendly with everyone, but friends with no one.

Fairness does not mean you have to pay everyone the same amount. You can have different pay rates, depending on skill level or other factors. You can also consider seniority for determining such things as vacation schedules.

Honesty speaks for itself. You must be scrupulously honest with your staff. Always tell them the truth. Never, never lie to them or try to cheat them in any manner. Bend over backwards to give them the benefit of any doubt in any situation in which you are not absolutely sure you're right. Even if you are sure, weigh any evidence to the contrary carefully. If the employee makes a good case for his or her position, accept the facts.

Make sure your employees have ample opportunity to earn a decent living. Remember why they're there. They work because they want to make money, not because they like you or because your salon is a happy, fun place to be. If they don't make money, they will leave and try somewhere else. To keep your employees, keep them busy. Make sure they are fully booked. This is why you shouldn't overstaff. Compensate them fairly and give them incentives to increase their bookings or production. Provide training that will let them expand their knowledge and skills and enable them to earn even more.

The Employee Handbook

Consistency is important, because it prevents surprises and employees always know what to expect from you. It means minimizing variables in your attitudes and in your dealings with the staff. Consistency starts with your Employee Handbook.

Developing an Employee Handbook is important. This is the manual that describes and defines your salon policies and practices. The exercise does two things for you. First, it makes you think about your policies and practices and put them in writing. Second, it formalizes those policies and practices and makes them easier to enforce. It should tell the employee everything he or she needs to know about working conditions in the salon.

CHECKLIST 10-2
ELEMENTS OF THE EMPLOYEE HANDBOOK

The Employee Handbook should contain:

1. Mission statement
2. Salon goals
3. Hours of operation
4. Services offered
5. History of the salon
6. Expected attitudes
7. Dress code
8. Expected conduct
9. Pay policies
10. Benefits
11. Disciplinary procedures
12. Any other factor relevant to the employees

The Employee Handbook should contain anything of relevance. It should include, but not necessarily be limited to, the following. Include your mission statement and your goals for the salon. Put in your hours of operation, the services you offer, and a brief history of the salon, if you have one. Give the employees a picture of the salon's background and its aims. Describe the attitudes you expect from each employee, toward their clients and toward each other. Establish your dress code, if you're going to have one. Define pay policies, such as when employees will be paid (weekly or monthly), how they will be paid (cash or check), and what will be withheld. Describe benefit policies, such as length and scheduling of vacations, vacation pay, and sick leave. Also, make sure to include your procedures for disciplining employees. This can be very important if you have to terminate a staff member.

Enforce the provisions contained in your handbook equally among all of the employees. Remember, they are the policies you've established and represent your view of how you want to run your salon. Any exception you make for one employee, you will have to make for all of them. You can revise your Employee Handbook as the need arises. Don't hesitate to make changes as your policies evolve.

But you need to formalize those changes by writing them down and making them applicable to everyone in the salon. When you do make changes, be sure the employees know about them. In fact, it's a good idea to discuss proposed changes, and the reasons for making them, with the employees before you proceed. Get their input. They may have some good ideas that you can incorporate. Plus, you'll help make them feel part of the team by giving them a voice in setting the policies.

Take the time and effort to develop your Employee Handbook properly. Think carefully about the information you put in it. Some of the provisions it contains may be considered as an implied contract, so before you issue it to employees, let your attorney review it.

Salary Compensation

There are three basic methods of salary compensation. You can pay an employee a salary, a commission only, or a combination of salary plus commission. Each has advantages and disadvantages for both you and the employee. In your salon, you will probably use all three methods, depending on the various positions.

A salary is a fixed wage, which can be paid on an hourly basis, for example, $6.00 per hour, or on some other time period, for example, $250 per week. For the employee, the advantage of this arrangement is a guaranteed amount of pay, regardless of the number of clients serviced, as long as he or she works the requisite number of hours. The disadvantage is that the employee has little or no opportunity to increase the amount. The advantage for you is that you have a fixed expense that will not increase even if the employee is extremely busy. Your disadvantage is that you are paying the same salary even if the employee is not busy at all. Plus, you have little incentive to offer to the employee. But you can have the employee perform other tasks, such as stocking shelves or sweeping the floor, when he or she isn't busy. If you intend doing this, however, make sure there is a statement in the job description that makes such duties part of the job.

A commission is an agreed-upon share of the amount of money the employee brings into the salon. For example, suppose your esthetician gets a 50 percent commission. Thus, if he or she performs $700 in services on clients in a given week, his or her pay will be $350. The commission percentage may be based on the total amount of the service, or on the amount after deducting the cost of materials. So, for example, if your esthetician gives a facial for $35.00 and the cost of the materials used is $5.00, the commission can be either $17.50 or $15.00. Whichever commission calculation method you use, make sure the employee knows the basis for the calculation right from the beginning.

The advantage of a commission to the employee is that his or her income is limited only by the amount of business he or she can bring into the salon. Theoretically, there is no upper limit. The disadvantage, on the other hand, is just the opposite. It is possible to have no income at all. The advantage to you is that you have no salary expense unless the employee has generated income. The amount you have to pay is directly determined by the amount the employee brings in. Your disadvantage is that you lose a measure of control over the employee. It is very difficult to have an employee on commission perform other tasks in the salon when he or she isn't busy. It is also more difficult to keep the employee satisfied during slow periods. To offset this disadvantage, you may offer the employee a draw, that is, an amount of money you pay during slow periods, which is deducted from future commissions when the employee is busy.

In the salary plus commission form of compensation, the employee receives a fixed wage, plus a commission on any amount exceeding a base figure. For example, the employee might receive a salary of $200 per week, and get a 40 percent commission on any amount he or she brings in over $400. Thus, if he or she performs $800 in services to clients in a given week, the pay will be $200 plus $160 in commissions.

This form of compensation combines the advantages of both of the other forms, with few of the disadvantages. The employee has a guaranteed minimum income, with an incentive to work harder and earn even more. You have the advantage of limiting your fixed salary expense while keeping the employee more content. You also maintain better control over the employee's time.

In part, the type of salary compensation you choose to pay each employee will depend on the negotiations between you and the employee. In part, it will depend on the particular needs and duties of the position. So, for example, you will probably pay your receptionist a salary, because he or she has little or no opportunity to earn additional income in the form of tips. Nor does he or she influence the number of clients who come into the salon. Similarly, you may pay a newly graduated esthetician a salary until he or she can build a clientele that warrants another form of salary compensation.

On the other hand, you may pay your more experienced cosmetologists on a salary plus commission basis or on a straight commission basis. Your best cosmetologists, who have large followings, may
want to receive only a straight commission.

Minimum Wage Laws

The Fair Labor Standards Act, passed originally in 1938, established
standards for minimum wages and overtime payments. The law is
enforced by the Wage and Hour Division of the Department of Labor.
As an employer, you are obligated to pay your employees at least that
minimum rate and must pay them overtime wages, calculated at time
and one-half their pay rate, for any hours worked past forty hours in
any one week.

Under the provisions of the wage and hour law, you may consider tips as part of the minimum wage as long as the amount of tips
is less than 40 percent of the minimum wage. You may not deduct for
the cost of tools or uniforms from your employees' regular pay if that
deduction causes the pay to go below the minimum wage.

Not all small businesses are covered under this law, so check
with your local wage and hour office to see if you are exempt from the
provisions of the law.

Tips, Bonuses, and Other Pay

Besides salary, there are other types of payment. These include tips,
bonuses, and benefits such as vacation, holiday, and sick pay. Except
for tips, these payments are exempt from wage and hour laws.

Tips make up a considerable portion of income for many salon
employees. As an employer, you should be happy to see your
technicians getting good tips. It will help keep them happy and
productive. More importantly, it means your clients are satisfied with
the services they're receiving. If an employee is not getting much in
tips, investigate the reasons. You may find areas for improvement,
either in the salon practices or in his or her work habits.

Bonuses are also an important form of compensation. They are a
reward for a job well done, and have a tremendous motivational
effect. If an employee performs over and above duty, or offers a sug-
gestion that improves the profitability of the salon, reward him or her
with a cash payment. If your salon does well, share the success with
your employees. After all, they are largely responsible for the success.

A bonus does not have to be large. Even small payments can go a long way, provided the employee recognizes why he or she is getting the bonus. Don't overdo bonuses, however. Their motivational effect can be diluted if they are so frequent that employees begin to expect them as a regular part of their pay. Establish sound fiscal parameters for bonus awards. And make sure they are applicable to all of your employees equally. Consult with your accountant to set these policies. But, be sure to take advantage of the benefit to you that this benefit to your employees can have.

Vacation, holiday, and sick pay are benefits that represent a reasonably small expense to you, but offer considerable benefit in keeping your employees happy. Offer your employees a paid vacation. In the case of salaried employees, base the amount on the weekly wages. For commission or salary plus commission employees, base the amount on the average weekly income. You can base vacation length on seniority, for example, one week vacation after one year employment, two weeks after three years.

Vacations and vacation pay are not regulated by wage and hour laws, so you have a lot of leeway in how you administer them. But remember fairness in both pay and scheduling. In a busy salon with many employees, scheduling of vacations is important. You don't want too many employees out at one time, so establish an equitable schedule, based on seniority. Set up a calendar at the beginning of the year. Your employees with the longest service get the first pick, and go on down the line until everyone has picked his or her weeks. Once the schedule is set, stick to it. You may let employees trade weeks among themselves, but make sure you are adequately staffed at all times. Of course, if you close the salon for a vacation period, all employees will take their vacations then.

Also, consider giving your employees paid holidays. Even though the salon is closed, pay the employees what they would have made that day, exclusive of tips. If the salon is open on a holiday, consider paying the employees who work that day at time-and-one-half. Consider also, giving each employee an extra holiday, such as getting his or her birthday off with pay. Again, the extra expense involved should be more than offset by the improved relationship with your employees.

Establish a policy for sick pay. If an employee is ill, pay him or her at the normal rate. You can set a limit, for example, six days per year. Any absences beyond that are not paid. Conversely, consider offering employees a small cash reward if they take no sick days in the course of the year.

Benefits

Salary is not the only form of compensation. To compete for good employees in today's job market, you have to offer a decent benefit package. Vacation, holiday, and sick pay are only a part of that package. There are many benefits you can offer that will make your salon a more attractive place to work in, not all of which have to be fully funded by the salon. There are a number of benefits you can offer for which the employees pay part of the cost.

Any benefit that enhances the security of your employees is a positive asset. For most employees, security for them and their families is a concern that ranks behind only the ability to earn a decent living. Life and health insurance plans meet this need, so think seriously about offering them. There are a number of plans available, through a variety of insurers. Some trade associations offer group health insurance plans, as well. Check with your insurance agent and your trade association for costs and requirements. With most plans, you can choose either to pay the full costs for your employees, or have them share in the cost through payroll deductions.

Pension plans are other benefits that provide security to employees. As with insurance plans, there are a number of different types of pension plans that you can set up. Some require you to contribute all of the funds; others allow employee contribution. Most have tax benefits for you and the employee, but also must meet strict IRS requirements and require complex record keeping and reporting. Simplified employee pension plans (SEPs) offer good benefits for the small business owner and employees and are free from much of the regulatory pressure of other plans. Your accountant, your insurance agent, or your banker will be able to advise you on costs and requirements of the various plans and will be able to help you choose the appropriate plan for your business. In addition, information is available in the Small Business Administration's booklet, *SEPs, What a Small Business Needs to Know*. The IRS also offers a number of publications explaining various pension plans.

There are two other benefits that offer particular advantages to salons, an industry in which the employees are predominately female.

To attract experienced cosmetologists who may have left the business to care for their families, you might lure them back to work by offering flexible hours or help with daycare for their children. Flexible hours cost you nothing. Daycare help, however, can be expensive, so check with a number of daycare centers to find the best value. Keep in mind you have to offer the benefits to all employees. You can't discriminate.

Training

Providing educational opportunities for your employees to enhance their skills can also be a benefit for you as well as them. The more highly skilled your employees are, the more income and goodwill they can generate for the salon. It also helps them make more money. For example, if one of your estheticians becomes an expert in lymphatic drainage massage, he or she can give therapeutic massage treatments. You expand your list of services, and the esthetician gets more clients.

Establish a training policy, using a combination of in-house programs and external courses. You might, for example, have a VCR and television monitor in the employee lunchroom. Keep video training tapes, which are available on a variety of subjects, on hand for them to watch. Keep a shelf of reference books on skin and body care techniques, and encourage the staff members to read them.

Hold monthly supplier nights, where you have a supplier or industry expert make a presentation on new skin and body care techniques. Many suppliers will be happy to do this. Have the sessions after closing hours or on a day the salon is closed. Provide light refreshments and make it a pleasant social occasion as well as an educational event.

Also, have your employees attend industry trade shows and seminars. Pay their admission fees and expenses. Get them involved in the activities of the local chapter of your trade association. Encourage them to attend the meetings and serve on committees.

You can also send your employees back to school for advanced training. For example, if you have an esthetician who you feel would make a good electrologist, send him or her for advanced training at the salon's expense. The additional income he or she can generate should more than pay for the schooling, as long as you utilize that extra training. Be careful with this, though. If you are paying for extra training, you want that employee to stay in your employ. So, you should have some kind of binding contractual agreement that he or she cannot quit and go to another salon for a specified period of time after the training, or must reimburse you for the cost, if he or she does leave. Ask your attorney about such contractual arrangements.

FIRING EMPLOYEES

Personnel management has its ugly side. Sooner or later, you will have to fire an employee. This is one of the hardest tasks you will face. No one likes to fire a staff member. It is a devastating experience for both sides. It is not easy to terminate someone, either from an emotional standpoint or on legal grounds.

Emotionally, you will feel a sense of failure that you were unable to motivate the employee properly, were incapable of getting better performance from the person, and made a mistake in judgment in hiring that person in the first place. You will feel some concern about that person's well-being, especially if he or she has a family. And you will feel sadness that such a step was necessary. You will have these feelings even though you may be totally blameless. These emotions are natural in decent, caring human beings.

You should understand, however, that sometimes it is necessary to fire an unproductive or badly behaved employee. A bad employee will cost you money, both through loss of customers and on the demotivating effect he or she will have on the other employees. Don't make the decision to fire someone lightly. Be sure of the facts and make the decision unemotionally. But, once you've made the decision, do it quickly. Letting a bad situation drag on does not make it any easier.

The emotional drain of the experience may cause you to lose only sleep. Inattention to the legal implications, however, can cost you hard cash. The general legal concept that influences employer/employee relations is the idea of "at-will" employment. This means that, unless there is a written contract that spells out terms of employment, the employee can quit anytime he or she wants, and you can fire the employee anytime you want. In practice, however, it is not quite that simple. Your ability to fire without cause may be limited.

One of the limitations may be the language you used in your salon information kit, your Employee Handbook, on your application form, or in the verbal comments you made during the interview. Anything you say or put in print may be considered by the courts to be an implied contract, and you can be held to those provisions. For example, when you made the job offer, did you say it would be a permanent position? The courts may hold that you promised the employee a job for life and will not be able to fire him or her no matter what the cause. Never offer anyone a permanent position. Offer a full-time position instead. This is why you must be careful what you promise and why you should have your lawyer review all written and printed documents that have anything to do with your employment practices.

No firing will be totally unexpected. There will be warnings—customer complaints, complaints from other employees, mistakes made, subtle changes in the employee's attitude and work habits. You should be aware of these and monitor what's going on in your salon. This gives you time to counsel the employee and take corrective action before firing becomes necessary. Make sure the employee has clear guidelines for the job and has a clear understanding of your expectations for doing that job. You have a lot of time and effort invested in the employee. Take every measure to correct a bad situation first. Termination should be your last resort.

Act on serious problems immediately. Don't let a situation build until it gets out of control. If someone is not performing adequately, let him or her know about it right away, and give him or her an opportunity to improve the performance. Prescribe a corrective course of action for the employee to follow, then track his or her progress in solving the problem. Make sure you talk to the employee privately, and keep the discussion confidential. Remember the rule—compliment in public; criticize in private.

Document all of the discussions you have with the employee. Write a detailed account of what you discussed and what conclusions you and the employee reached. Give a copy to the employee and put a copy in his or her personnel records. Note especially if the employee has acknowledged the problem or has denied having difficulty. Document your follow-up actions, as well.

Performance Reviews

You can catch a lot of problems early by giving each employee periodic performance reviews. These should be private, formal sessions held on a quarterly, semi-annual, or annual basis, in which you and the employee discuss his or her progress and performance. This is a two-way process, so give the employee an opportunity to talk and to evaluate his or her own performance. This is a time to identify any less serious problems and take steps to correct them.

Include your performance review policy in the Employee Handbook. Place a written record of each review in the employee's personnel records. The performance review should not be held only to discuss problems. Use it to point out what the employee is doing well and to reinforce good performance. The review should be a positive experience.

Disciplinary Procedures

Your salon should have a formal, written procedure for disciplining employees that should be included in the Employee Handbook. The procedure should spell out the reasons for discipline and how it will be carried out, and it should be followed equally for all employees.

The procedure should spell out in detail the steps involved, starting with warnings, moving to probation or suspension, and leading to termination. There is no legal requirement to give an employee warnings or to put him or her on probation before firing, but if you have such procedures described in your established policy, make sure you adhere to them. Have your attorney review your disciplinary procedures. As with anything else involving employees, document each step as it occurs and keep a complete record in the employee's file.

The Firing

Once you have exhausted all corrective measures and have reached the decision to terminate the employee, carry it out immediately. Call the employee into the office and tell him or her. State truthfully and clearly why he or she is being let go, and go over the evidence leading to the decision. Make your offer of severance pay and explain the employee's rights to collect unemployment compensation. You have no legal obligation to offer severance pay, but the employee may be entitled to collect unemployment benefits if he or she was terminated for incompetence or for lack of work. If the employee is fired for cause, that is, for actions such as insubordination, theft, or nastiness to customers, he or she may not be entitled to those payments. You can ask your state department of labor for guidelines about employee eligibility for compensation.

Have a third party in the room as a witness. Record the employee's reaction and response to the firing. Document the event and keep copies. Do not get into an argument over the firing and don't change your mind. If you have followed your disciplinary procedures, have issued warnings, and have tried corrective actions, the firing should not be a complete surprise to the employee. Have the employee collect his or her personal belongings and leave the premises immediately.

The fired employee will probably apply for a job in another salon and may use you as a reference. If another prospective employer calls you to check that reference, be very careful. You can verify the dates the person worked for you and what his or her duties were. Do not go into details of why the person left your employ or give any derogatory information. This could leave you vulnerable to a later lawsuit.

Also, let your other employees know that you have fired this person. You do not have to tell them why, nor should you. The details are not their business. You should reassure them, however, that the firing was an isolated incident and that their jobs are safe.

When you are able, examine the events that led to the firing. Do this objectively and dispassionately and learn from the experience. Were your expectations and guidelines clear enough? Could you change your interview and audition procedures to identify problems before you hire a person? What steps can you take to avoid having similar problems with other employees?

Good personnel management is vital to your business. It is time consuming and difficult, but important to your success. Do what's necessary to find, motivate, and keep good employees. When you've made a mistake and have hired someone who doesn't work out, don't be afraid to terminate him or her. Establish sound personnel management principles and follow them. Keep careful records and you should be able to minimize your problems.

SUMMARY

How well you hire and train employees will be a major factor in the success or failure of your salon. It is difficult to run a business without having competent employees on whom you can rely. You will probably need a number of employees, filling positions that let you provide the services you offer in your salon. Make sure you hire enough employees to meet your needs; however, you should be careful not to hire more employees than you need.

Employees are not your only concern. You will also need to work with a number of independent contractors, such as your accountant, your attorney, and cleaning services. While these people perform services for you, they do not work for you, so you are not responsible for withholding taxes or providing benefits. Be aware of the various taxes you must consider on behalf of your employees. It is necessary to keep meticulous records of all employee transactions.

Finding good employees is a difficult task; keeping them is more difficult. It is important that you make your salon an inviting place in which to work, both to attract help and to keep their loyalty. To help you, develop a salon information package that describes your salon and your business philosophies, and details the benefits an employee will get by working for you.

There are a number of sources for finding employees. You can advertise in the help-wanted section of the newspapers, utilize employment agencies and job placement services, or solicit employees from other salons. You might also rely on your current employees to recruit qualified people they know. The local beauty school may also be a good source of new employees for entry level positions.

When hiring, conduct interviews and auditions carefully. This is the stage when you will find out all you can about the prospective employee. Examine resumes closely and check references. Be aware of the legal implications of the process, however. Once you have made a decision, make the hiring offer. Make sure all the terms of employment are clearly understood by the person. Keep a written record of all agreements. Establish a probationary period for the new employee.

To keep employees, be fair, honest, and consistent at all times. Have firm salon policies, written in an employee handbook, and make sure all employees adhere to them.

One of the most difficult tasks you'll face is firing an employee, but it is sometimes necessary. No matter how careful you are in the hiring practice, you will sooner or later hire someone who does not work out. When you fire someone, however, be very aware of the legal implications. You can save yourself a lot of trouble by conducting regular periodic performance reviews of your employees. This is a way to catch problems early and take steps to correct them. Make sure you have written, formal discipline procedures, and follow them equally with all employees.

After you have exhausted all other remedies and decide that firing is necessary, don't hesitate. Do it quickly and in private. Have a third party as a witness and document everything.

EQUIPMENT AND SUPPLY MANAGEMENT

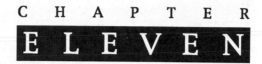

ELEVEN

In the course of operating your business, you will need a large variety of equipment and supplies. These are of many types, such as the machinery and materials you use to provide the services you offer, the equipment and supplies you use to run the administrative functions of the business, the chemicals and hardware you use to clean and maintain your salon, and the retail products you offer for sale.

Regardless of the type of equipment and supplies you use in your salon, remember one thing. They all cost money and represent an expense. Their purchase and use must be managed, the same as every other aspect of your business. How well you manage your equipment and supplies will have a direct effect on the profitability of your salon. Manage these assets poorly and they will be a constant drain on your resources. Manage them well and they will pay for themselves many times over.

Review the discussion on cash flow in Chapter 9. Cash flow is the difference between income and disbursement. You will have to spend money to purchase supplies, so you must have enough cash available to let you buy those things that make money for you. If you overbuy or buy the wrong things, that unused and unneeded stock ties up the cash you may require to buy supplies or services you really need. And that can cost you both business and money if you don't have the materials you need to service your customers and don't have

the resources to get them. You need to make sure you have sufficient
funds to meet your needs. As stated earlier, if you run out of cash,
you go out of business. Don't waste your cash on things you don't
need right now.

EQUIPMENT

Equipment refers to those items of machinery, fixtures, and furniture
that you purchase or lease only once and which have a long life span.
These include capitalized items whose costs you can amortize over a
given period of time and can depreciate on your tax returns. They
include such items as skin care machinery, facial chairs, manicure
tables, computers, and cash registers (Figure 11-1). Noncapital equipment includes tools, such as scissors, electrology needles, and ventouses, that are purchased seldom and have a reasonably long life span.
These are treated as a one-time expense on your tax returns, in the year
in which they are purchased, and are not depreciated over time.

The type of equipment you need will depend on the services you
offer. (Specific equipment requirements are discussed in Chapter 4.)
Obtain equipment only as you need it. Don't overequip your salon.
Equipment that sits idle costs you money, both in the actual dollars
you spend and in the loss of those funds for other, perhaps more
important uses. Keep your equipment working and generating
income for your salon. You can always add more equipment when
you have a real need for it. But, make sure you have enough equipment to service your customers adequately. You have to strike a
balance. That means you have to stay on top of your business, so you
always know what is going on in your salon.

Regardless of the type of equipment you need, make sure it is the
best quality you can afford. Top-quality equipment, even though it
may cost more originally, is actually a better investment. It works
more efficiently and lets you do a better job. It lasts longer than cheap
equipment, and it looks more professional. The quality of the equipment you get will tell your prospective clients a lot about the quality
of the services you offer.

Purchasing Equipment

There are many manufacturers of good-quality skin and body care
salon equipment. You can find them through their advertising in

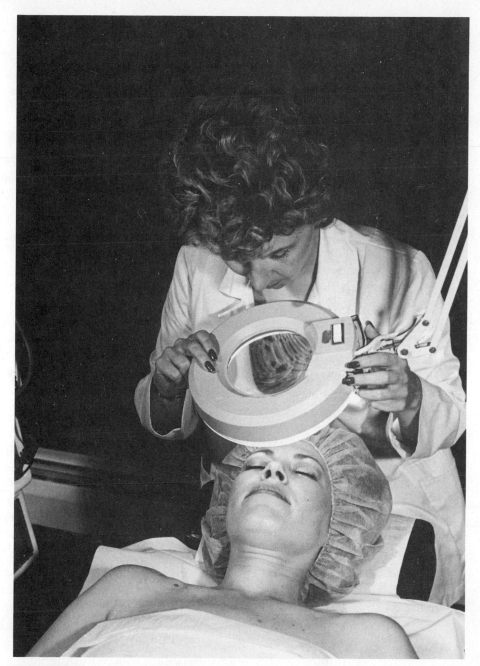

FIGURE 11-1   Magnifying lamp

major cosmetology trade magazines, through demonstrations at industry trade shows and exhibits, and at your local salon supply distributor. Call or write to these companies and get their catalogs, price lists, and distributor locations. Examine the catalogs and pick the equipment that best suits your needs. Whenever possible, look at and try out the actual equipment before you make your final decision. Then negotiate your purchase (Figure 11-2).

Don't be afraid to shop for the best deal and don't rush into an equipment purchase. Take your time. Investigate all of the factors involved to be sure you make the right choice. Don't consider only price. You may be able to negotiate for a better price, but you won't get it unless you ask for it. Look also for extra costs, such as shipping or set up charges. Do you have to pay for delivery or does the manufacturer include that cost in the price? Does the equipment require any accessories you will have to purchase before you can use it in your salon? Many times the price of the unit may be fixed, but the extra charges will be negotiable. It is often possible to negotiate terms, too. Instead of paying the entire price up front, you may be able to pay in thirty, sixty or ninety days. This lets you put that money to work for that time and effectively reduces the cost of the unit. Or you might be able to negotiate payment on monthly or quarterly terms.

Check the guarantee or warranty on the equipment. How long is it? Just what does it cover? Look also for service. Who will provide maintenance or repairs on the equipment? Will it come from the manufacturer or the distributor? Will the seller lend you a replacement unit if yours is out for repair? Does the manufacturer provide training on the unit? For example, some manufacturers of skin care machinery hold free training classes in the proper use of their equipment. Service is a very important consideration with equipment. You may be better off buying from the supplier who gives the best service, even if the price is slightly higher. In this competitive age, you'll probably find that all manufacturers charge roughly the same prices for comparable equipment. All things being relatively equal, base your decision on superior service. This concept shouldn't come as a surprise. The superior service you offer to your clients could be the determining factor in their decision to patronize your salon.

You may also consider purchasing used equipment. It is often possible to get good deals on pre-owned gear, which may be on the market for a variety of reasons. Salons go out of business, remodel, or

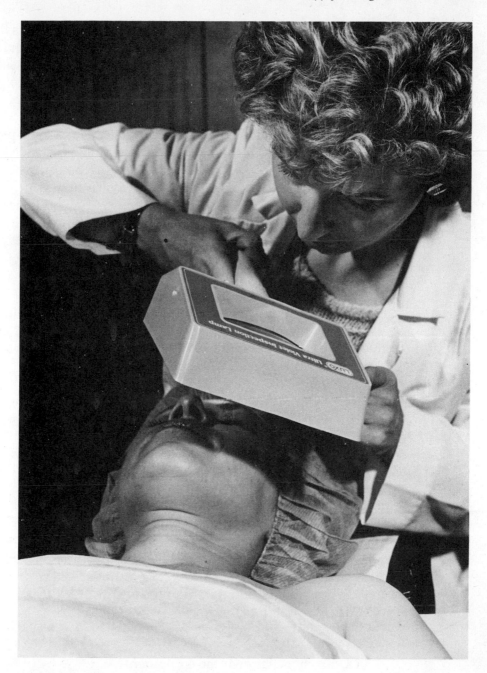

FIGURE 11-2   Wood's lamp

change their mix of services so the equipment no longer suits their needs. Whatever the reason for its sale, that piece of used equipment may be a good buy for you. Make it a habit to check the classified advertising section of your daily newspapers and trade magazines. Look over used equipment offerings at your local salon supply distributor when you are there for other purchases.

When you buy used equipment, you should take some precautions, however. Know what comparable equipment costs when new, so you can determine a fair price for the used machinery. Look it over carefully. Does it match your salon decor? Will it fit in with your other equipment? Do you really need it now or can you foresee a need for it in the near future? As with any equipment, if it sits idle in your salon, it is no bargain.

Check the equipment's condition. Is it in good repair, both operationally and cosmetically? Does everything work properly? Are all the parts present? Will it require any repair or refurbishment before you can use it? What will it cost to repair or refurbish? Is there still a valid manufacturer's warranty on the equipment, or will the seller give you a guarantee? If you're buying the equipment directly from a salon

CHECKLIST 11-1
BUYING USED EQUIPMENT

1. Know what comparable equipment costs when new.
2. Does it match the salon decor?
3. Is it in good condition?
4. Are all parts present?
5. Does it need any repair or refurbishment?
6. How much will repairs cost?
7. Is the equipment still under the manufacturer's warranty?
8. Can you get a written guarantee from the seller?
9. When was the equipment purchased?
10. How was it used?
11. Why is it being sold?
12. Examine the original invoices and paperwork.
13. Does the seller own the equipment?
14. Is it currently collateral for loans?
15. Negotiate the price.

that is going out of business, you're not likely to get a guarantee from the seller. If you buy the used equipment from a broker, however, you should get one. In any case, ask for a guarantee, and get it in writing.

Ask questions. When was the equipment purchased? How often was it used? How was it used? Why is it for sale? Did the seller buy it new or used? From whom? Does the seller have the original invoices and paperwork? If so, examine them. These papers will verify the age of the equipment and tell you how much the seller paid for it.

There's another very important point, although it might sound like a simple question. Ask if the seller owns the equipment. Does he or she have clear title to the equipment and have the authority to sell it? If the seller still owes money on the equipment, or if it is pledged as collateral for a loan, you may find yourself liable for paying those debts, or you may lose the equipment. Get a written statement from the seller that he or she has clear title to the equipment. This will give you some ability to recover your money if the seller has sold it to you fraudulently, although realistically your chances of ever getting that money back are slim, especially if the seller has declared bankruptcy and gone out of business.

Keep in mind when you negotiate the price of used equipment, that you may be able to get an even better bargain if the seller still owes money on it. You might be able to get it for very little cash, just by assuming the remaining payments. Just make sure that the total for the cash plus the rest of the payments is less than the cost you would have paid if the seller owned it free and clear.

Leasing Equipment

You may also be able to lease some of the equipment rather than purchase it. Leasing offers some financial and operational advantages. Financially, leasing may be advantageous because you don't tie up large amounts of cash up front. You pay, instead, a fixed monthly or quarterly fee for the use of the equipment for the length of the lease period. You do not incur a debt, such as you would have if you borrowed the money to buy the equipment, so you may find it easier to obtain a bank loan. In addition, you may have some tax benefit, since you can treat the lease payment as a business expense and deduct it from your income taxes, instead of depreciating the equipment over time. Discuss this point with your accountant. Since there is no longer an investment tax credit for leasing equipment, the actual tax benefit you might get will vary from case to case.

From an operational standpoint, leasing has the advantage of giving you more flexibility in maintaining and upgrading the equipment. As new, more efficient equipment becomes available, you have the ability to exchange your older models for state-of-the-art models. You won't be stuck with obsolete equipment.

One disadvantage of leasing is that you have no equity in the equipment. At the end of the lease period, you don't own it unless you have negotiated a purchase provision as part of the lease agreement. Since you have no equity in the equipment, you can't use it as collateral for business loans. Another disadvantage is that you have limited flexibility during the term of the lease. If you want to cancel the lease before it expires, you may incur significant cost penalties. If you go out of business while the lease is in force, you may be held personally responsible for the remaining payments.

Employee Tools and Equipment

One significant factor you will have to determine is how you will handle the tools and equipment used by your employees. Will you supply everything they need to work, or will you require them to supply their own? Your decision will become an important part of your salon's policy. It should be included in your Employee Handbook and be enforced equally for all employees.

You will supply all of the major, large fixed pieces of equipment, such as facial chairs and skin care machinery. Since these pieces of equipment must match your overall decor, it is unreasonable to expect the employees to furnish them. You may, however, require them to supply their own personal tools. Your advantage here is that you don't bear either initial or replacement cost of these items. Also, your cosmetologists will usually be more comfortable handling their own tools, which they will be more used to, and will generally take better care of them, since they will have to replace the tools when they wear out.

The disadvantage of this policy is that you lose some measure of control over the quality and design of the tools they bring to work. You may find it difficult to insist they purchase and use a particular brand or style of equipment, and this may have an adverse effect on your overall decor. In cases such as this, you may find it desirable to supply the tools yourself.

So decide your policy carefully. Where the style and type of tools matter, supply the equipment for the technicians. Where it doesn't matter, have your employees use their own tools, as long as they are of suitable quality. You can suggest they have certain tools. Keep track of tools you supply and insist the employees take reasonable care of them.

SUPPLIES

Supplies are those items you use on a regular basis in the course of your business operations, and which are generally used up in the course of business. Unlike tools and equipment, they have a relatively short life span and are purchased on a recurring basis. They may be categorized, in general terms, as reusable, disposable, and consumable. Reusable supplies are items that are used repeatedly including towels and smocks, which are used, washed, sterilized, and made ready for reuse. Disposable items are those that are used once and discarded, such as cotton pads and disposable bonnets. Consumable supplies are those that are used up during use, such as cleansers, toners, and masks.

The division of equipment and supplies into such specific categories may seem questionable, but these are important distinctions. Thinking of these items in this way will force you to think more like a business person and will enable you to keep track of your expenses and to allocate charges more accurately. It will help you determine the true costs of your services and help you stay competitive. It will also help when you fill out your tax returns.

You will require many different types of supplies to operate your business. You can categorize these as operational supplies, administrative and office supplies, maintenance supplies, and retail sales goods. All are important. Like your equipment, your supplies all represent a significant business expense that must be managed properly to maintain your profitability. The following discussion of supply requirements is not meant to be comprehensive. It is virtually impossible to list every conceivable kind of product you will need in your operation. The discussion is meant only to spur your thinking about your needs and to demonstrate the vast scope of the subject.

Operational Supplies

Operational supplies are those items you use to provide the services you offer. They are utilized by your cosmetologists in the course of the workday. The exact supplies you need will depend on the services you offer. If you offer complete skin care services, for example, your consumable supplies will include a variety of cleansers, toners, astringents, facial masks, and moisturizers for different skin types (Figure 11-3). Disposable supplies will include lancets, cotton, gauze, hair bonnets and spatulas. Reusable supplies include towels, blankets, and drapes. For waxing services, you will need wax and body lotions as consumables, muslin strips and paper sheeting as disposables, and towels and drapes as reusables.

Consumable supplies for manicuring include polish removers, assorted colors of polish, nail tips, and acrylic nail materials. Disposables include cotton, emery boards, and orangewood sticks. For makeup application you'll need consumables such as various types of cosmetics and cleansers; disposables such as cotton balls, swabs, and head covers; and reusables such as towels and drapes.

As you can see, the list is seemingly endless. But each item has an important place in your business. You must be aware of every item you need, regardless of its size or cost.

Administrative and Office Supplies

Administrative and office supplies are used to accomplish the business functions other than the services you offer. These include your business letterhead stationery and envelopes, business cards, appointment books, appointment cards, ledgers and other bookkeeping supplies, pencils, pens, staples, and paperclips. They also include file folders as well as various forms you use for employment applications, customer files, and employee records.

In this category, you can also consider items you need for your reception area, such as magazines, styrofoam cups, coffee, tea, cream, sugar, and stirrers. Your supply requirements in this area, though of different types, are no less important than your operational supplies.

Maintenance Supplies

Maintenance supplies are used to clean and maintain the facilities and the equipment. They include various cleaners and disinfectants used to clean the floors, walls, windows, and mirrors; mops, brooms, and

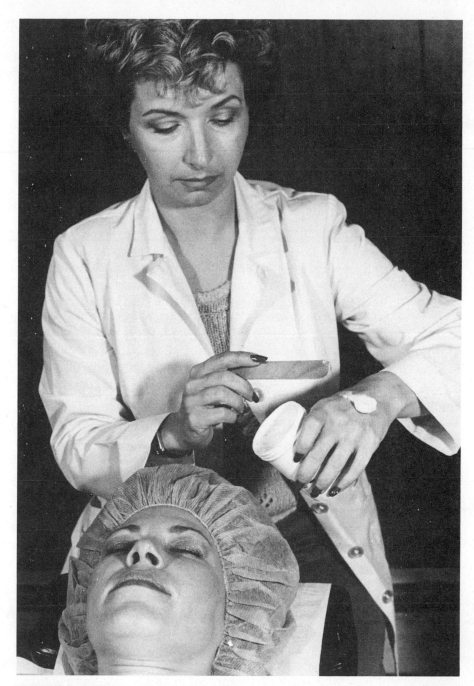

FIGURE 11-3 Cleanser use

buckets; and alcohols and chemicals used to clean and sanitize your implements. Don't forget items such as extra fuses and spare light-bulbs, either. You might also include in this category, those items you need for your rest room facilities, such as hand soap, toilet tissue, and paper towels.

Retail Goods and Supplies

Retail goods and supplies are those products you offer for sale to your clients as well as the materials you need to help you sell those goods. (Retailing and the materials needed are discussed in Chapter 13.)

PURCHASING SUPPLIES

Purchase your supplies with the same care and consideration you utilize to buy your equipment. Many of the same principles apply. Investigate your purchases thoroughly, and buy only what you need. Consider service as well as price. Choose your suppliers carefully, and don't be in a hurry to buy anything.

Determining Supply Requirements

To determine your supply requirements you need to ask two questions. What products do I need? What quantities of those products do I need? Note the emphasis on need. Get only the products that enable you to keep your salon operating and enhance your profitability. Anything else is a waste of your resources. Also, buy only for your immediate needs, not for something you might do or require in the future. When it's time to get those items, you can acquire them.

The types of products you need will depend on the services you offer (Figure 11-4). Each service, whether skin, body, or nails, has its own supply requirements. You should know what they are, if you are competent to offer the service. Before you buy an item, make sure you know what you will use it for—your operations, your office, or retail sale.

You have a wide choice of product lines, or brands, from which to choose. In your salon, you may use either name brand or generic products. Which you purchase will depend partly on the type of salon you operate and the clientele you service. If you operate a high-volume, budget-priced salon, for example, you may want to use only the lower priced generic materials for your services. Conversely, if

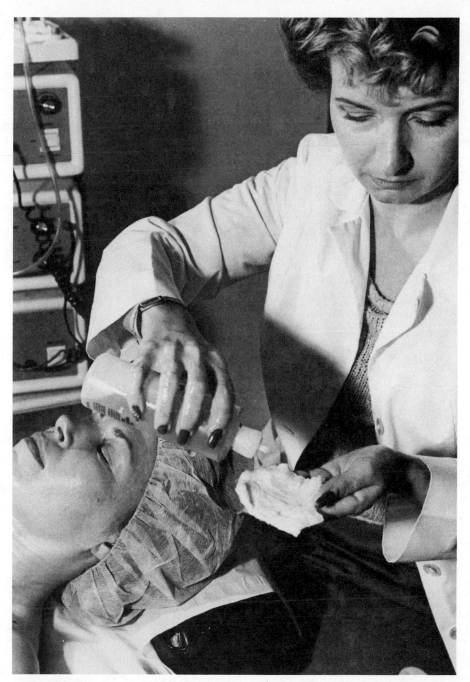

FIGURE 11-4   Toner use

you service primarily affluent clients and command high prices for your services, you will want to use the more expensive name brand products. In actual practice, you will probably use a mix of both—the less expensive generic products where their use won't adversely affect your image; the costlier name brands where it makes a difference.

If you sell products at retail, you should use those same products in your operations. It is very difficult to convince your client to spend $20.00 on an eight-ounce bottle of name brand skin cleanser if you've just treated his or her skin with a $5.00 bottle of generic cleanser.

Whatever products you buy, however, whether generic or name brand, make sure they are of the best quality (Figure 11-5). Quality products are important to your services. You can't do first-rate work with second-rate materials. Like equipment, good-quality products are a better investment than poor-quality products, even though they may cost more. They will usually do the job better and lead to better customer satisfaction.

Quality varies from one product to another, even among name brands, and though brands may have comparable quality, one may suit your operations and your ways of working better. Also, not all of the products in a manufacturer's line are necessarily of the same quality level. You might find, for example, that manufacturer A has the best cleansers, but its masks are of lesser quality, while manufacturer B has outstanding masks but not such good cleansers. You don't have to limit your selection to one brand, so feel free to mix and match. Choose those products that you're comfortable with and that work best for you, even if they are from different manufacturers. However, don't overdo the mixing and matching. Limit the number of brands you utilize to keep your inventory control manageable.

Test all products thoroughly before you buy them in your normal quantities. Make sure they work for you, through actual experience in your salon under the conditions you face. Read the manufacturer's instructions and any available literature about the products thoroughly. And follow the manufacturer's instructions. They are there for a reason. Know the ingredients of every product you use and know what role each ingredient plays in the product. Get Material Safety Data Sheets (MSDS), available from the manufacturers on request, for any product that might be classed as hazardous, for example, hydrogen peroxide and acetone. If you don't understand any part of the instructions or the contents, ask the supplier. Don't use a product unless you understand its composition and use thoroughly.

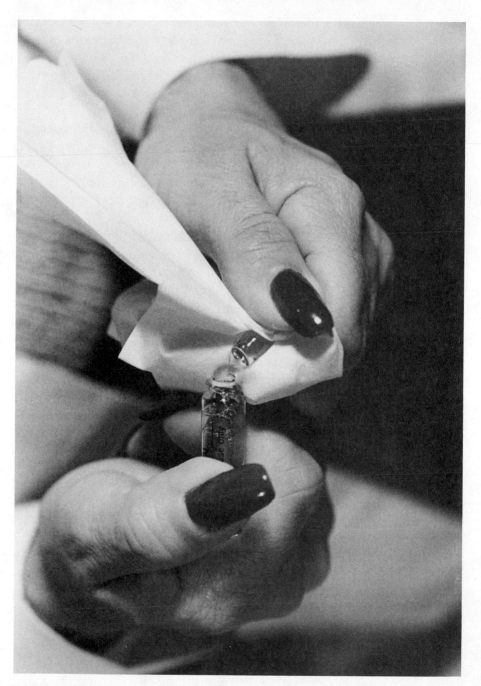

FIGURE 11-5 Ampoule use

Keep a file on every product you use or sell in your salon. Include the MSDS forms and complete specifications in the file. Keep notes on the performance of each product, especially if you experience a problem with it, and keep these in the permanent record as well. Review the notes periodically to see if there are any changes in the performance of the product. Also review the ingredients periodically to be aware of any changes in the composition of the product. If there are, ask the manufacturer why the change was made. Become so familiar with the products you use that you can answer any question clients may ask about them. Remember, the clients view you as the expert in the field. Make sure you don't disappoint them through lack of product knowledge.

Your job doesn't end once you've made your product selections. You must stay abreast of new developments in the field and be aware of new product introductions. When you see a new product, test and evaluate it to see if it might earn a place in your salon. When you find a better product, don't be afraid to make a change. Just make sure you change for a good reason.

New products are often introduced at regional and national cosmetology trade shows, and are usually described in the beauty industry trade journals. Attend shows and read the journals. Get all the information you can. Even if you decide a new product is not suitable for your salon, you should still be aware of its existence and its properties. You may not be interested in a new product, but some of your customers may be, so you should have enough information to answer at least basic questions about the product.

Many factors go into your product decision. Quality, of course, is mandatory. If the product is of low quality, any price is too expensive, no matter how low it is. Reliability is also important. Does the product perform adequately? Does it do what it is supposed to do, and does it do it consistently? If you can't rely on the product, it is not good for you. Suitability is a concern. Does the product meet your needs? Are you comfortable with it? Does it fit the way you do business? If it isn't suitable, it's not a good buy. Don't discount service, either. Does the manufacturer or the supplier stand behind the product? Can you count on delivery when you need it? And then there's price. Don't base your purchase decision on price alone. Consider price only when everything else is equal. You should be more concerned with value, which is the sum total of all of the factors.

Determining Supply Quantities

Once you've decided on the products you will utilize in your salon, you must determine the quantities of each you will purchase and stock. If you are just starting in business, this can be difficult. It is easier when you've been in operation for some time and have developed a business history.

The object is to strike a balance so that you have a large enough quantity of each type of supply to meet your immediate needs, yet not so much of each in inventory that you're tying up your cash needlessly or that the materials pass their expiration dates before you can use them. Don't overbuy. Excess inventory is a waste of valuable resources. The only possible justification for buying more of a particular product than you need for reasonable immediate use is if you get an especially good deal, such as a special sale, or if there is a significant discount in the price for buying in larger quantities. Even then, be careful. Make sure you will still use the product within a reasonable amount of time. Analyze the situation on a case-by-case basis. Be certain that the amount of money you will save on the sale outweighs the loss of ready cash you may need for other uses.

The quantity of any given product you should buy depends on two factors, the frequency with which you perform the services in which it is used and the ease with which you can replace the product. Once you've been in operation for awhile, if you have kept adequate records, you will be able to predict how many times you will perform a service in a given time period.

Suppose, for example, when you analyze your records you see that your salon averages fifteen facials, eight makeovers, fourteen body wax treatments, and twelve manicures each week. Based on these statistics, you can determine how many of each service you can reasonably expect to perform in any given week. You know how much product it takes to perform each service. Multiply the average number of services by the quantity of product used for each to give you a base quantity requirement for each product. You can consider this number as your minimum quantity requirement.

Statistics, however, give you only an average, not an absolute number. They don't account for variations in your business due to seasonality, holidays, or special promotions you may offer, so you must add a safety factor to your minimum quantity to account for increased business in any given time period. So, for example, if your base quantity of dry skin cleanser is seven units, you might want to establish a normal stock quantity level at ten to twelve units, and a maximum stock level at fifteen units. This means, then, that for this cleanser, your reorder point will be seven units and you will not keep more than fifteen units in stock, unless you have a special promotion on facials that may require more inventory.

Go through this exercise with each product you use. Establish minimum, normal, and maximum stock levels for each. Once you've done this, monitor those levels constantly and adjust them as necessary. You may adjust your maximum stock level according to how easy or difficult it is to replace the product. If you can get the product quickly from a local beauty supply distributor, you can afford to have a lower maximum stock level. If you must order the product from a distant source and wait for delivery, you might want to have a higher maximum.

Note that this discussion is based on a careful analysis of your business. If you are just starting your salon, you will not have this data available and that will complicate your decisions. In this case, you must make some basic assumptions about the level of business you will enjoy and base your stock level decisions on those estimates. Make your assumptions realistic and err on the side of caution. Here, you will probably be better off by underbuying until you have a more accurate feel for your business. Adjust your supply purchases as you acquire more information.

SUPPLIER RELATIONSHIPS

The Supply Pipeline

Before you choose your suppliers, you should understand the supply pipeline, which consists of the manufacturer, distributor, wholesaler, retailer, and end user. The manufacturer makes the product. Although the manufacturer may sell the product directly to the end user, more often he or she sells it to a distributor, who warehouses the product and sells it, in turn, to a wholesaler. In many cases, the distributor is also a wholesaler. The wholesaler sells it to the retailer, who then sells it to the end user. The retailer may also be the end user. This is the case in the salon. You are both the retailer, for those products you sell to your clients, and the end user, for the products you utilize in providing the services. The local beauty supply store, where you will purchase many of the supplies, is the wholesaler. The store can get its stock either from the distributor or directly from the manufacturer.

The distributor, wholesaler, and retailer are the conduits through which the manufacturer gets the product into the marketplace and to the end user. At each step, the number of people handling the product gets larger and the quantities of the product get smaller. Thus, the manufacturer, a single entity, makes the product in a huge quantity. Smaller portions of that quantity go to a limited number of distributors around the nation. Each distributor further breaks down the quantity and sells a smaller number of units to a larger number of wholesalers. Each wholesaler continues the process, selling a smaller number of units to a larger number of retailers. At each stage, the pipe gets smaller but has more branches.

The price of the product increases as each handler in the pipeline adds a markup to the cost. The manufacturer sells the product to the distributor at a price determined by the product's cost of research and development, raw materials, manufacturing, packaging, and administration expenses, plus a profit. The distributor adds a markup based on his costs plus profit. The wholesaler does the same, and so does the retailer. The consumer pays the highest price. When you use the product in your service, you figure the cost of the product into the price of the service, so even here, you are passing that cost on to the consumer.

At each stage, though, the quantities of the product involved decrease as the unit price increases. As an illustration of the cascading price and diminishing quantities, consider this example. Assume each handler adds a markup of 40 percent. Suppose you sell a client 1 eight-ounce bottle of Brand A toner for $10.00. You purchased 6 bottles from the wholesaler at a cost of $7.14 each. Your 40 percent markup is $2.86. That is not your profit. You have to consider your costs of doing business into that figure. The wholesaler purchased six cases (72 bottles) of the product at $5.10 per bottle. The 40 percent markup here is $2.04. The distributor purchased six hundred cases (7,200 bottles) at $3.64 each. The 40 percent markup here is $1.46. The manufacturer produced sixty thousand cases (720,000 bottles) at a cost of $2.60 per bottle. The 40 percent markup here is $1.04.

Note also, that as prices rise and quantities diminish, the risk diminishes. If the product turns out to be unsaleable, you are only stuck with 6 bottles and are out $42.84. The manufacturer is stuck with 720,000 bottles and is out $1,872,000.

As a general rule, the higher up the pipeline you can purchase the product, the less you should have to pay for it. If you can buy directly from the manufacturer, you should save a considerable amount, although you won't get a price as low as a distributor would pay, simply because you won't be able to buy the product in the same large volume as a distributor. Some manufacturers will not sell products on a direct basis.

Choosing a Supplier

It is important to establish and maintain good relationships with your suppliers. A good supplier does more than just sell you products. He or she should also be able to provide you with a wide range of services and information. Choose your suppliers with the same care and consideration you use to pick anyone with whom you work.

You will undoubtedly purchase your supplies from a number of sources. Different suppliers handle different types of products and different product lines. However, you should limit the number of suppliers you work with. Have more than one supplier for each type of product so you have an alternative source. That way, if one supplier can't supply the immediate need, you have somewhere else to turn. But don't have too many suppliers, either, as that weakens any relationships you establish. Two to three suppliers for any given type of product should be sufficient.

Most of the products you purchase will probably come from your local beauty supply wholesaler, although you may also purchase some items directly from the manufacturer. Each source offers advantages and disadvantages. When you buy direct, you eliminate part of the supply pipeline and may get a more advantageous price. In addition, you open a direct channel of communication with the manufacturer and have a better opportunity to ask questions and gather more information about the product and its uses. However, your choices will be limited by the manufacturer's product line offerings. Obviously, you can only buy the products the manufacturer makes. Your orders will be made by mail or telephone and you will have to wait for delivery. It is more difficult to establish a good working relationship with a manufacturer so your dealings will be more impersonal.

In contrast, your beauty supply wholesaler offers a much wider range of products, produced by a large number of manufacturers. While you may place orders by mail and telephone, most wholesalers have store locations where you can pick up your supplies. This eliminates the wait and lets you reduce the quantities of the products you have to keep in inventory. You get faster service and can develop a relationship with the wholesaler. The disadvantage is that you are farther along the supply pipeline and prices may be somewhat higher.

Check out all of the suppliers within a reasonable distance from your salon. Visit them and talk to the managers. Ask questions. See what products they handle. Do the suppliers stock the products you want to use? Is the stock fresh? Are the stores clean and tidy? Are the salespeople knowledgeable? Do you get personal attention? What other services do the suppliers offer—training classes, product demonstrations, free delivery? Do the wholesalers seem to be reliable? What payment terms are offered? Do you always have to visit the store location to purchase your supplies, or do they have salespeople who will call on you? Do the suppliers stand behind the products they sell? Are their prices competitive?

Do the suppliers sell only to salons, or do they also compete with the salons by selling the same products to consumers? Some beauty salon supply outlets sell only to licensed cosmetologists. Others, however, will sell the same salon grade products to consumers. This practice undercuts your business since it competes, often unfairly, with your salon. Some manufacturers sell their products directly to consumers, which also gives you unneeded competition. When you can, purchase your products only from suppliers who support the beauty industry and who don't try to make a profit at your expense.

From your initial survey, choose the suppliers with whom you're comfortable and begin to establish a working relationship with them. Get to know the people and let them get to know you. Let them know that you intend to do a significant percentage of your business with them, but let them know, also, that they have to earn it. You are their customer and deserve the same treatment your customers expect from you. Discuss your needs and requirements and make sure your expectations are clear.

Don't choose your suppliers on price alone. Look for service and quality as well. Reliability is important. You have to be able to trust the suppliers to get you the products you need when you need them. The best price is useless if you can't get the goods on time.

By the same token, they can expect you to be a good customer. Be fair in your dealings with the suppliers. Don't make unreasonable demands or play one supplier against another. Treat the suppliers the way you want your customers to treat you. Remember, they are entitled to make a reasonable profit, too. Be loyal to your suppliers as long as they provide the products and service you require. If they stop meeting your needs, by all means look for new sources. But don't hop from one supplier to another just in search of the best price.

Cash Versus Credit

When you are first starting with a supplier, you probably will purchase your supplies on a cash basis. This will hold true especially if you are just starting in business. Once you've built a relationship you may be able to purchase on credit terms. If you can, by all means do so. Let your money work for you. But, make sure you pay your bills on time. If you get thirty days to pay, make sure you pay the bill within that time, but don't pay earlier unless you get a discount.

Your invoice may contain terms such as 2%10, net 30. This means that you can take a 2 percent discount from the total if you pay within ten days, but must pay the total amount if you take the full thirty days. If possible, take the discount and pay within the stated time limit. Given the relatively small invoice amounts and short time periods involved, the discount amount will usually be greater than the amount of interest that the money would earn if you left it in the bank for thirty days. The discount adds to your profit.

INVENTORY CONTROL AND MANAGEMENT

It is important to establish strict controls over your inventory, which must be managed just as all other aspects of your business. Inventory is money. Each item you stock costs real dollars. If these items are lost, stolen, or misused, it means money out of your pocket.

In a busy salon, it is easy to lose track of products. With the hustle and bustle of everyday operations, it is sometimes hard to devote the time and effort to monitor such a seemingly simple operation as inventory control. You can forget to log incoming products or neglect to record products you use. Either way, you lose track of them and can't figure where they went. That represents lost money.

No matter how honest you think your employees and your clients may be, it is a hard fact of life that some people steal. Products may be stolen from your inventory easily unless you take precautions. Stolen or misappropriated products also mean lost money.

Waste is another profit robber. When products are misused, spilled, ruined, or pass their expiration date, they can't be used to earn income for you. Wasted products are wasted money.

Don't make the mistake of thinking that at most you'll only lose a few small items and that the cost will be insignificant. A trickle can soon become a flood that will drown your profitability and ruin your business. Institute sound inventory handling practices right from the start. Know where every item that comes into your salon goes and how it is used. That means more than buying the right products in the appropriate quantities. It also means storing the goods securely, controlling access to them, and keeping accurate and up-to-date records.

Inventory security starts from the moment you receive the goods into the salon, extends through their storage, and ends when you use the product and discard the empty package. When products are received, don't leave them unattended. If you haven't the time right then to log them in, put them in a secure area until you can. Then log them in as soon as you can, but certainly not later than the end of that business day. Don't put them into your stock until they are logged in.

Whenever you receive an order, count every item. Match what you received against the invoice to be sure you get everything you ordered. If the order is short, notify the supplier immediately. Don't pay for goods not received. If items are backordered, ask the supplier when they will be delivered. You don't have to pay for backordered items until you receive them.

Keep your inventory in a locked supply room or in locked cabinets if you haven't a suitable room to use for the purpose. Know where the keys are at all times. Only employees should be allowed in the supply room, and you may want to limit access to certain ones. As part of your salon procedures, establish who will have the authority to take products from the inventory. Have anyone who takes a product out of the room sign it out, recording his or her name and the date. This is not just for security purposes. It also lets you monitor your business activity.

Organize your supply room so that products are easy to locate. Keep similar products together. Keep the room well lit, clean, and uncluttered. Arrange the stock so that the oldest products are taken first. Be aware of the expiration dates of all products and use them before that date. Discard any product that has passed its expiration date and remove it from your inventory. Dispose of the outdated products properly. If you are purchasing the right products in the right quantities, you should not have too many products that go out-of-date. If you see a pattern developing, adjust your purchases accordingly.

Set up an inventory control card for each product type. The card should contain the name of the product, the minimum and maximum quantities that you have determined for it, and the amount on hand. The minimum quantity is the reorder point for the product. Whenever a product is removed from the room, whoever takes it should sign and date the card. The card should stay in the area in which the product type is stored.

Set up a product log, as well. This is your primary record of your supply purchases and use. Record every product that comes into the salon. Record the date received, the quantity and price, and the supplier. Then note in the log every time you use a product. This is an ideal function for a computer. Keep a running inventory with your supply log. In addition, conduct a physical inventory periodically. (You may want to do this quarterly.) Note any differences between the physical inventory and your running inventory. This is an indication of product shrinkage and may be due to theft, loss, or waste. Try to account for all discrepancies.

Don't just keep records; analyze them. They are another business tool that helps you maintain profitability. Accurate records show you patterns of business. They let you utilize your supplies in the most efficient manner and get the most for your money.

SUMMARY

Equipment and supplies are necessary to the successful operation of your salon. They cost money and so represent an expense for you. Just as any expense, they must be managed properly to prevent an adverse effect on your profitability.

Equipment refers to the machinery, fixtures, and furniture that have a long life span. The services you offer will determine the type and quantity of equipment you'll need. Buy only what you need. Unused equipment only ties up capital and doesn't generate income. But make sure you get the best quality equipment you can afford.

Shop for the best deal on equipment. There are many sources for most types of skin and body care machinery, furniture, and store fixtures. The equipment may be either new or used, but be especially careful when buying used equipment. In some instances, you may find it preferable to lease the equipment.

Supplies are those items that you use in the day-to-day operations of the salon. They may be reusable or disposable. Either way, however, they have a relatively short life span. There are different types of supplies. Operational supplies are those used to provide the services. Administrative and office supplies are those used in the business aspects of the salon. Maintenance supplies are those used in cleaning and repair of the facilities. Retail supplies are those intended for resale.

Purchase supplies with the same care and attention to detail as you use when purchasing equipment. Like equipment, supplies represent an expense. Buy only what you need to operate for a reasonable time. Don't keep excess inventory. That only ties up your capital. Whatever products you buy, however, make sure they are the best quality you can afford. Establish an inventory control system to keep track of all supplies. Keep records on supply use and analyze those records periodically to develop data on use patterns that will help you manage your supplies effectively.

Establish good relationships with your suppliers. Check what other services and information the supplier can provide for you. Always be honest with your suppliers, and pay your bills on time. Don't buy just on price; look for quality and service, too.

CHAPTER
TWELVE

Your salon's operations, the policies and practices you follow in your day-to-day business, are critical to your success. How well you run your salon can make or break your business. You are operating a service business in a highly competitive field. To succeed, you need to follow three rules:

1. **Satisfy the customer.**
2. **Satisfy the customer.**
3. **Satisfy the customer.**

It is impossible to overstate the necessity for keeping your customers satisfied. Without following this one not-so-simple principle, you have no business and nothing else you do will matter.

Pay attention to the "three Cs" of successful salon management: competency, consistency, and consideration. From your customers' point of view, competency means that the services and products you provide are of the highest quality, are performed quickly and efficiently, and are done to the customers' complete satisfaction. They feel they have received the best value for the money they've spent. Remember, your customer, not you, determines quality. From your point of view, competency means that you handle all the aspects of your business to the best of your ability.

Consistency means that your customers know they can rely on you and your employees to do the job right every time they patronize your salon. It means you are open when you're supposed to be open, you have the services available when they're supposed to be available, and your salon never wavers in the quality of the services it provides. In short, it means you are reliable.

Consideration means that you treat everyone with respect—your customers, your employees, and the people with whom you do business. Your honesty is above reproach. You operate your salon under the most stringent ethical standards, recognize the value of a good reputation, and do what you must to earn it. You understand that your customers are the reason for your business and you pass that understanding along to your employees. You go out of your way to make customers feel appreciated, thereby earning their respect and patronage.

CUSTOMER RELATIONS

It's easy to satisfy your customers. All you have to do is give them what they want at a reasonable price in a comfortable setting in a manner that makes them feel they've been treated honestly and fairly and have received an outstanding value. Satisfy your customers and you will keep them. Fail to satisfy them and you won't. It is as simple as that. It's the key to repeat business.

First, you have to know what they want. That means you have to know what you're selling. Understand the differences between the features and the benefits of your services. The service is what you offer; its features are its identifiable attributes; its benefits are what it does for the client. There is a very definite distinction here. You may think you're selling the features, but you're not. The clients may think they are buying the service, but they're not. They are buying the benefits of that service, even though they may not realize it. That's what you should be selling.

For example, consider a basic facial. That is the service you are offering. The features of that service include cleansing the skin, normalizing its function and protecting it. The benefit of the service is that it makes the client look and feel good. When your clients come into the salon, they don't want a facial but want to look and feel better. If you don't understand that difference, you'll have a hard time satisfying them. If your clients believe they look and feel better when they leave your salon, they will come back. If they don't, they won't, no matter how technically perfect the facial may have been.

There are other factors to consider in customer satisfaction as well. You have to treat clients with courtesy and appreciation. All clients are guests in your salon. You have to provide surroundings that make them feel comfortable and confident. It is important to establish an ambience in your salon that reinforces the trust and confidence you expect your clients to have in your business. A skin and body care salon, more than most businesses, relies on a bond of trust between the clients and the people who provide those services. Without that bond, the clients will never feel as though they've been really satisfied.

Your objective is to build customer loyalty to your salon, and to have repeat business. You need to keep those customers coming to you over and over again. It is easier and less expensive to keep customers than it is to continually find new ones. Building a solid base of satisfied clients is the key to your business success, and, you want them to be loyal to the salon, not necessarily to any particular employee. You want customers to stay, even if the esthetician they always utilize leaves. This is extremely difficult. The beauty business is very personal and intimate and clients build close relationships with their cosmetologists. You have to offer them a reason to stay with you. That reason starts with the way they are treated in your salon and the degree of satisfaction you provide.

Ideal Clients

Ideal clients know what they want and make those wants known clearly. They are on time for appointments and cooperate with the technicians who perform the services. These clients are friendly and fair, expect to be completely satisfied, and will not accept anything less, but do not make unreasonable demands. Ideal clients are very easy to deal with. Unfortunately, not all clients are ideal.

In the course of your business, you will encounter many different kinds of clients, who may be insecure, angry, dissatisfied, late, rude, demanding, impossible, or a combination of any or all of these. Some may be very difficult to deal with. No matter how trying clients may be, however, you must treat them with the same competency, courtesy, tact, and restraint with which you treat all other clients. It is an axiom in business that the customer is always right. This is especially true in a service business. So remember that the customer is always right, even when he or she is wrong.

This does not mean that you have to be a doormat or compromise your principles. You should be polite, accommodating, and fair, but you must also be firm. Never lose your temper or argue with clients. Stand your ground with courtesy and dignity. No matter what the provocation, stay calm and collected. Give clients the benefit of the doubt. Instill these same qualities in your employees.

Insecure Clients

Insecure clients don't quite know what they want and aren't sure of their needs or of your ability to fill them. With this type, you need to be patient and reassuring. Spend a little extra time to get to know about them. Explain everything you do and be encouraging, but be careful not to be patronizing.

Angry Clients

Angry clients are upset at something. Recognize that their anger may have nothing to do with your salon. With this type, stay calm and cool. Find out why they are angry. If it is because of something that happened in the salon, assure them you will do something about it. Empathize and be conciliatory. Apologize if necessary, but don't get into an argument. Try to have your discussions in private so a scene does not develop in front of other customers or employees.

Dissatisfied Clients

Dissatisfied clients have a complaint about some aspect of the service. Find out the source of the dissatisfaction, and offer to correct the problem. Again, be conciliatory and fair. Don't argue with these clients. You may win the argument but lose the business. Don't do anything that causes clients to lose their dignity. But be firm if the complaint is not valid. State your position calmly and stick to the facts, then negotiate a compromise. One of the most important points to remember here is to listen and be sympathetic. Many times, that's all that may be necessary.

You should encourage your clients to complain to you if they are not satisfied. If there is a problem, you want to know about it and take steps to correct it. A dissatisfied customer who doesn't complain is a lost customer. Statistics show that up to 96 percent of unhappy customers don't complain to the business. But they do complain to as many as ten other people. And the noncomplainers are not likely to come back to your salon. By the same token, clients who do complain to you are likely to come back, even if their complaint has not been completely resolved.

Late Clients

Late clients always show up late for appointments. Any client may be late on occasion. You can usually work around that. Chronically late clients, however, can be a major problem for you and are very disruptive to your business. They can throw off your entire schedule and cause your cosmetologists to run late, which creates severe problems for your other clients, who are unfairly forced to wait. You must be polite but firm with these clients. Explain the problem they cause. If they are more than fifteen minutes late, cancel their appointment and offer to fit them in when you can or reschedule. Be aware that if you take this stand, you may lose these clients. But be aware also that if you don't, you may lose many other clients—who won't necessarily complain to you. They'll just stop coming.

Rude Clients

Rude clients are always nasty and pushy and can be a real challenge to work with. You cannot be rude or nasty back. Be polite, even though it may be difficult, and don't take the rudeness personally. Remember, it is part of their personality. They have to live with it; you don't. Perform your services quickly and well, and get these clients in and out of your salon with a minimum of fuss. Be alert, however. Don't let their demeanors disrupt the activities of your salon.

Clients can have bad days and experience rude streaks. Clients who are normally nice may, on occasion, be nasty. In this case, a casual conversation should uncover the cause of the problem. Empathize and treat them with friendliness and kindness. Once they are calmed down, they will probably revert to a normal personality and may even apologize for the nastiness.

Demanding Clients

Demanding clients can be especially difficult to work with. They are very exacting and insist on having things their way, right now; know exactly what they want, even when it may be wrong; and often make unreasonable demands and unjustified complaints. Remember that many times, clients who make unreasonable demands know they're unreasonable and don't expect you to accede to them. All they really expect is to get some smaller compromise.

Stay calm. Don't argue or lose your temper. Be polite, but be firm. State your position and stick to the facts. Compromise when you can. If you are totally justified, however, don't be afraid to say no. This is hard to do, but once you give in to an unreasonable demand, you leave yourself open to even more outrageous ones.

Occasionally you will have clients who insist on services that you know will not be suitable for them. Now, you face a dilemma. If you give them what they want, they won't be satisfied and will be angry. But if you refuse, they'll be dissatisfied and angry. Remember the distinctions discussed earlier about what you're selling. You know that what these clients really want is to look good. That fact plus your expertise are your answers. Explain the consequences to be faced if you give what has been requested. Make sure they understand those consequences. Show how unhappy they will be with the results, and convince them to rely on your professional experience and skill.

If clients still insist on receiving a service after all your discussion, you have two choices. You can either perform the service or you can refuse. Either way, you face the loss of clients. Let your integrity and professionalism be your guide. You may be better off by suggesting they get the service in another salon. If they go elsewhere and are unhappy, at least they'll be unhappy with the other salon, and may even realize you were right after all and come back.

Always keep in mind that you are the professional. If you perform an unsuitable service at a client's insistence, especially if you know the service may damage the client's skin, you can be held liable for that damage, even though a release may have been signed. If you know damage may occur, refuse to perform the service.

Impossible Clients

Impossible clients combine the worst traits of all of the previously discussed types. They are unreasonably demanding, rude, selfish, inconsiderate, and constantly complain about everything. They upset your employees and annoy your other customers. No matter what you do, you cannot satisfy these clients. With this type you must still be courteous, but you must also be firm. Decide whether you really need their business. You may be better off without it. If they are disruptive, suggest they take their business elsewhere. Don't let these people drive away other clients and cost you business.

You will also face other problem clients. In the course of your business you will encounter customers who come in drunk, drugged, disorderly, dirty, or diseased. State laws prohibit you from working on clients who have a contagious or communicable disease. Follow the law. Suggest that these clients see a qualified physician and come back when they are better. Do not perform services on these clients. The same holds for clients who come in dirty or with bugs. Again, do not perform services on them. You can insist that clients be physically clean before you work on them. Don't let them infect your salon. Abide by sanitation laws.

Drunk, drugged, or disorderly patrons can only disrupt your salon's decorum and operations. Refuse service to anyone who fits this category. Be courteous but firm in dealing with them. Don't argue or let them disrupt your salon. If they will not leave peaceably, call the police and have them removed.

Handicapped Clients

Handicapped clients are not a problem. As customers, they are just as valuable as able-bodied clients, but may require special consideration. Federal and state laws prohibit discrimination in service because of disabilities. Handicapped individuals have special needs that you must consider, most often involving access. Make sure your salon is accessible to the handicapped. That means doorways that are wide enough to accommodate wheelchairs as well as rest room facilities that are suitable. Consult your local Equal Employment Opportunities Commission (EEOC) office for specific requirements for handicapped access.

Your handicapped clients deserve the same courtesy, consideration, and competence that you extend to your other clients. Go out of your way to accommodate their special needs. Recognize their limitations and work around them. Above all, however, don't be patronizing. Be aware of any medical conditions they may have that preclude specific services, for example, massage or use of electrical apparatus during a facial. If you have any doubt about the safety of a service, check with their physicians.

CHECKLIST 12-1
SALON POLICY MANUAL

Your Salon Policy Manual should contain the following:

1. Salon hours—days and times of operation
2. Pricing—all services consistently priced with the prices posted
3. Rules of employee conduct
   A. Attitudes toward customers
   B. Attitudes toward each other
   C. Dress codes
   D. Food and beverage handling in the salon
   E. Gum chewing
   F. Smoking
4. Scheduling appointments—lateness policy
5. Payment for services—cash, check, credit cards
6. Use of the telephone—for business only

SALON POLICY AND PROCEDURE MANUAL

Consistency demands that you establish sound, written policies and procedures for your salon. Create a policy manual that states these clearly. Make sure all of your employees are aware of the policies and abide by them. This can be part of the Employee Handbook discussed in Chapter 10. You should abide by these policies, too.

SALON HOURS

Have a definite schedule for your salon. Establish your opening and closing hours and days of operation, and post them in a conspicuous place in the salon. Be consistent. Be open and ready for business when you're supposed to be. Your customers should be able to rely on those hours. If you are going to close the salon for vacation, make sure your customers know the dates far in advance. This might sound like a simple policy, but it is often ignored. It can be hard to fight the temptation to close the salon early on a day that business may be light, but don't do this. If you deviate from your set and posted hours, you will develop a reputation for unreliability.

   If you must close the salon for a short period because of some emergency, call all of your clients who have appointments and reschedule. Emergencies do happen and you have to be flexible enough to handle them. But make sure you only close in a real emergency when there is no other alternative.

PRICING

Establishing your prices is covered in Chapter 9. Whatever prices you set, display them conspicuously in the salon. Make sure your customers know the prices of the services when they come in. Be able to defend your prices if your customers question them. You know what your services are worth and what it costs you to perform them. Don't deviate from your price list by giving certain customers discounts. No matter how hard you try to keep it secret, your other customers will find out and will become alienated.

   You may on occasion have a special sale or promotion, which includes a price reduction on certain services, but keep these to a minimum and have a sound reason for taking such an action. Keep track of your costs and prices and adjust them, if necessary.

SALON AMBIENCE

Salon ambience is more than just the decor. It is the feeling the client gets when he or she walks into the salon. It is the atmosphere generated in the salon and should foster confidence and trust. Your salon should be bright, cheerful, clean, and inviting, and your employees should be friendly and courteous. Everything about the facilities and staff should make the client feel both welcome and appreciated. Colors, sounds, smells, and attitudes are all important. (Color use in salon decor is covered in Chapter 5.)

   With respect to sound, make sure there is no unneccessary noise in the salon. Choose the background music with care, according to the tastes of your clients, not of you or your staff. You may be the world's biggest rap music fan, but if the demographic analysis of your clientele shows they are into opera, you play opera. If in doubt about the type to play, stick to middle-of-the-road music. Don't turn your nose up at what some people disparagingly call "elevator music." It may not inspire anyone, but it won't offend anyone either. Whatever you play, keep it low. It should remain in the background and not intrude into the activities in the salon. Its purpose is to soothe and calm, not to entertain.

Salons generate certain smells. The various chemicals you use, manicuring supplies, for example, all have a distinct odor. You can't help that. But you should keep those odors to a minimum with proper ventilation. Use air fresheners where appropriate to keep your salon smelling good. Bad smells turn off clients. Remember, you may be so used to the odors that you don't notice them, but your clients will.

Attitude starts in the reception area. Was the client met with a cheerful welcome and a smile from the receptionist? Does he or she have a comfortable place to sit? Is there fresh coffee or tea available? Do you have a good stock of current magazines that are not dog-eared or torn?

Attitude continues in the working areas of the salon. Did the employees have a friendly greeting for the client? Did the service start within a few minutes of the appointment time? Was the client spared a long wait? Was the service done quickly, efficiently, and to the client's complete satisfaction? Did the technicians thank the client after the service? Did the cashier thank the client? Did you thank the client for his or her patronage? Did you ask how he or she liked the service? Did you ask whether he or she was satisfied? Did you let the client leave without being satisfied? Did you invite the client back?

EMPLOYEE DEMEANOR

You understand the importance of good customer relations. Make sure your employees understand that also. Your employees interact with your customers. Establish and enforce your rules of employee conduct, and make sure they are included in your Employee Handbook. Instill in your employees the necessity for courtesy and respect at all times. They should be friendly with customers, but not familiar. It is up to you to set the example for your employees. If you don't practice what you preach, you can't expect them to pay attention to your rules.

Maintain a professional image for your salon. You and your employees should look and act the part of professional cosmetologists.

Set a dress code according to the image you want your salon to project. Will it be casual? Trendy? Formal? That's up to you, but make sure the employees dress accordingly. Have your employees wear the latest hair and nail styles, too. You are selling the concept of looking and feeling good, so demonstrate it in your salon.

All of your employees should also respect each other and work together. They should be friendly and cooperate. When in the public areas of the salon, they should work in harmony. Keep internal disputes among your staff off the salon floor. Good-natured banter among the employees should be encouraged. Horseplay, however, should not be tolerated as it degrades the salon image and is dangerous.

Employees should be in the public areas of the salon only while working. Breaks and meals should be in the break room. Don't allow eating in the public areas of the salon. Whether to allow them to smoke in the public areas is a decision you'll have to make, but no smoking should be allowed in any of the treatment areas. Again, let the image you're projecting for your salon be your guide.

Inevitably a dispute will arise between an employee and a client. Be careful how you handle this. Both sides are important to you and you can't alienate either party. Don't automatically side with either. Stay impartial. Find out the facts and act accordingly. Conduct the discussion with both parties present and do it in your office, not on the salon floor. Be fair. If the issue is not clear cut, you may give the benefit of the doubt to the client, even if the employee is right. If you do, however, explain the reason to the employee, in private. If you've trained your employees in good customer relations, he or she will understand why you've taken the conciliatory action. If the employee is wrong, point out his or her mistake. Again, do it in private after the client has gone. Remember the golden rule of employee management: Compliment in public; correct in private. Stand behind your `employees and let them know you'll back them up when they are right and won't embarrass them when they make a mistake.

SCHEDULING AND APPOINTMENTS

You don't want to discourage walk-in business, particularly for new clients. All customers should be welcome. They all represent a source of income for your salon. But much of your business will be conducted by appointment. How you schedule and handle those appointments will be an important part of your customer service. When handled correctly, they contribute to customer satisfaction. When handled poorly, they can severely damage your business.

An appointment is nothing more than an agreed-upon, pre-arranged time for the customer to come into the salon and purchase one or more services. It is a commitment for both you and the client. The client has, in effect, promised that he or she will come in at a specific time for a specific service. You have promised that you will be ready to perform that service at that time. You have a right to expect the client to be prompt. By the same token, he or she has the right to expect to receive the services without undue waiting.

Honor those commitments. Unfortunately in many salons, the commitments are honored more in the breach than in the observance. That is a sure sign of poor management. Nothing will cause you to lose business faster than making your clients wait when they have an appointment and have come in on time. Some clients will just walk out. Some will complain but stay and wait. Some won't say anything at all. But they all will be aggravated and will stop coming back, no matter how good the services may be. And whether they complain to you or not, they will complain to many others outside your salon.

Making your clients wait shows great disrespect for them and disregard for their time. Remember, they have other things to do. They are busy people, too, and you're in business to serve their needs. They're not there to keep you in business. They represent your income, so you can't afford to lose customers because you've alienated them.

There are many reasons your scheduling can break down and appointments overlap. A client who has scheduled a leg waxing might decide to get a facial. Another client could be unavoidably late. Most clients understand that things happen unexpectedly and will accept having to wait on occasion, especially if they have been made aware of the problem and given the option of rescheduling or waiting, and the wait will be relatively short. Your problems start when you develop a pattern of making them wait almost everytime they come in. That is intolerable.

The receptionist should know the work schedule of each technician and what hours he or she will be available to receive clients. In addition the receptionist should be thoroughly aware of the capabilities of each technician and how long each takes to perform the various services, then use that information when booking the appointments. The object is to allow enough time to take care of the needs of each client but not to have too much idle time between appointments. Pacing is important. For example, if Mrs. Jones has a 9:00 A.M. appointment for a facial with Suzanne, and she takes one hour to do the job, you wouldn't schedule Suzanne's next appointment for 10:00. You would schedule it for 10:15, allowing enough time to clean the treatment room and get it ready for the next client. You can compress or expand the time needed as the conditions allow.

Of course, you should also consider the individual timing preferences of each cosmetologist. Just don't lose sight of the fact that the appointments are for the benefit of the client, not the staff. The object is to get the client in and out with a minimum of aggravation and a maximum of satisfaction.

Write down all appointments in a special log book you keep for that purpose. Enter a series of columns across the top of the page, one column for each cosmetologist. Enter the times in fifteen-minute increments down the left side of the page. Use a new page for each day. Beauty supply stores stock preprinted appointment books. Consider using one of these.

Log each appointment in the book as soon as it is made. Don't trust to memory. Enter the client's name, a telephone number where he or she can be reached, and the service to be performed in the appropriate time slot under the technician's name. Keep the book accessible to the technicians so they can check their schedules as needed. When you fill an appointment book, keep it as part of your records. The information it contains is a valuable cross reference for your other records.

THE RECEPTION DESK

The reception desk is the skin care salon's nerve center for scheduling appointments. It is one of the most vital areas in your salon, just as your receptionist is one of the most valuable members of your staff. How well it is operated has an effect on your business.

The receptionist is the first person your client sees on arrival and is the last person your client deals with on departure. The way the client is treated here sets the tone for the experience he or she has in your salon. The receptionist's effect on the client starts even before he or she comes into the salon. It starts with the initial telephone call.

In a busy salon, the receptionist may have many duties. The primary function of the position is to keep people and services moving smoothly by scheduling appointments effectively. He or she may also maintain your customer database, do basic bookkeeping entry, collect payment from the clients, keep the reception area in good order, and see to the needs of the clients before they are turned over to the technician.

The attitude your receptionist projects is important. He or she must have an outgoing personality, be friendly, courteous, and enjoy working with people. He or she should have the ability to keep smiling and stay pleasant, even when dealing with a difficult client. In addition, he or she should look the part, that is, be well dressed and groomed, with good posture and personal habits.

Training is essential. Make sure your receptionist is familiar with all of the salon procedures and practices, knows and practices good telephone techniques, knows about the services offered in the salon, and is aware of how long each cosmetologist takes to perform the services.

When the receptionist starts in the morning, he or she should review the appointments for the day and pull up the file on each customer who is due in. He or she should then brief the technicians on their schedules for the day and remind them of any relevant personal information about the clients coming in. Next, he or she should make sure the reception area is ready to receive clients.

As the day progresses, the receptionist should monitor the progress of the appointments and make sure everything is running on schedule. If a cosmetologist is running late, the receptionist should check with him or her to see if the time can be made up. If not, the receptionist should call that cosmetologist's remaining appointments and let them know there may be a delay, giving them the option of waiting or rescheduling the appointment.

As soon as a client comes into the salon, the receptionist should welcome him or her with a smile and greeting, recognition of the reason for the client's visit, and any appropriate information. For example, the conversation might go something like, "Good morning, Mrs. Jones. How are you today? I see you are getting a facial this morning. Suzanne will be with you in a moment. Would you like a cup of coffee?" Note what has happened with this exchange. The client has been greeted in a friendly manner, knows she is expected and that you are ready to serve her needs, and has been made to feel welcome. You have set the stage for a pleasant experience that will lead to her satisfaction and repeat business.

If the receptionist is busy on the phone making an appointment with another customer or conducting other business when the client comes in, he or she should still immediately acknowledge the client's presence, by saying for example, "Excuse me, I'll be with you in a moment." Then the client should be greeted properly as soon as the receptionist finishes the phone conversation. (It should go almost without saying that the receptionist should not be making a personal call when the client enters.)

All of this is just common courtesy and good manners, coupled with good business sense. The receptionist (as well as all staff members) must remember that the client is the reason he or she is earning a living and not an intrusion on their time.

When the client leaves, the receptionist should collect the payment if this is part of the duties of the position. In any case, he or she should thank the client, compliment him or her on the success of the service, ask if everything was satisfactory, and try to book the next appointment. He or she may also suggest that the client purchase products for home use. An appropriate conversation may go something like, "I hope you found everything to your liking, Mrs. Jones. Thank you for your business. We appreciate it very much. Can I make an appointment for you for your next visit? Good bye. We hope to see you again." You've made the client feel appreciated and you've let her know you want her continued business. The way she is treated when she leaves reinforces the mindset you tried to instill in her when she came in.

At the end of the day, the receptionist should gather all of the sales slips and match them with the appointment book to help the process of daily reconciliation. Before leaving the salon for the day, he or she should make sure the reception area is in good order.

THE TELEPHONE

The telephone is a valuable business tool, but unfortunately is also one of the most abused. Like any tool, it must be used properly. You should have a policy for telephone use, just as you do for any other tool in your salon, and you should train your staff in proper telephone procedures.

You certainly need a telephone at or near the reception desk. You may also want to put one in the salon office, possibly on a separate line. Consider your needs carefully. Have as many lines installed as you need to handle the amount of business you enjoy. Keep the salon phone strictly for business use. It should not be used for personal calls either by your staff or your clients. That telephone is one of your keys for bringing in business. Don't have it tied up by unnecessary incoming or outgoing calls, except in an emergency. Consider putting in a pay phone for customer and employee use.

You might also consider adding an 800-number service for your clients' convenience. This lets people call you on a toll-free number. The telephone companies have many 800-number service plans, designed specially for small businesses. Check with your telephone company for information about the service. If you do get an 800-number service, make sure you include that fact in your advertising and promotion. Many times, toll-free calls help bring in additional business.

How you and your staff answer the telephone is important. That phone call is, in many cases, the first contact customers have with the salon, and the way it is answered forms their first impressions. Again, remember common sense and courtesy. Answer the phone promptly, not later than the third ring. Waiting for someone to answer the phone is very high on the list of things that annoy clients. By the seventh ring, you've probably lost the business.

Watch your voice when you answer. Speak clearly and loud enough to be heard, but not too loud. Be friendly and courteous, and answer with a smile. Welcome the caller properly with an appropriate greeting, the salon name, and your name. For example, your receptionist might answer the telephone this way: "Good morning. ABC Salon. This is Jennie. How may I help you?" Answer with enthusiasm and warmth and never sound impatient. Don't just go through the motions. It will show, even without face-to-face contact. Never answer with a hurried "hello" or "yeah." Both are in bad taste and are bad for business. Before you answer the telephone, make sure you're composed and ready. Take a deep breath, relax, then pick up the phone.

Keep a notepad and pencil by the phone. Be ready to write down notes without delay. You may want to keep a telephone log, a record of all telephone calls. Get the caller's name and write it down. Keep it in front of you during the conversation so you can refer to it. When you reply, use the caller's name, as in "Mrs. Smith" or "Mr. Jones," but don't be overly familiar. Never use the customer's first name unless you have some indication that it will be acceptable to him or her. And make sure you get the name right; that's why you write it down. Don't be afraid to ask for the correct spelling.

Be ready to answer the customer's questions about your services or to book an appointment. Be responsive to the customer. When you book an appointment, ask what service the customer wants and whether he or she wants a specific technician. Consult the appointment book and negotiate an acceptable time. Make sure you allow enough time for the appointment. Get a telephone number where the client can be reached if there are any changes.

End the conversation by confirming any arrangements and thanking the caller. For example, you might say, "Okay, Mrs. Smith, we have you down for a facial with Suzanne on Thursday at 10:15. Thank you. We appreciate your business."

Don't put a caller on hold unless it's unavoidable. Even then, be careful not to leave the caller on hold for any length of time. If you have more than one telephone line and are in the midst of one call when the second line rings, excuse yourself to the first caller and put him or her on hold briefly. Then answer the second line, tell the caller that you will be back to him or her in a moment, go back to the first caller and finish the business. Apologize for the delay. Get back to the second caller as soon as possible and apologize for the delay again. Be composed, courteous, and friendly at all times, no matter how hectic the day may be.

You may want to have an answering machine for the times your salon is closed. Leave a simple message on it that gives your days and hours of operation, asks the caller to leave his or her name and telephone number, assures that someone will return the call, and thanks the caller. For example, the message might be, "Hello. ("Hello" is acceptable in this context) This is the ABC Salon. We are open Tuesday, Thursday, and Saturday from 9:00 A.M. to 6:00 P.M. and Wednesday and Friday from 9:00 A.M. to 9:00 P.M. At the tone, please leave your name and telephone number and someone will return your call. Thank you for calling." Check the answering machine for messages frequently and return the calls. Use the answering machine only when the salon is closed.

CASH AND CREDIT MANAGEMENT

You will have to decide whether you will run a cash only business or extend credit to your customers. You will also have to decide whether to accept personal checks. Cash is safer. When you extend credit, you always run the risk of not recovering the money. Plus, you risk losing a client when you apply vigorous collection methods. Credit also increases your bookkeeping load, especially with the relatively small amounts involved. With checks, you run the risk of nonpayment, plus it takes longer to get your money. As with credit, you may lose a customer if your collection efforts are vigorous. (But consider this: is it worthwhile to you to have a client who doesn't pay his or her bill?)

Handling Cash

At the beginning of the day, make sure you have enough cash in the till to make change. Have a supply of small bills, especially ones and fives, as well as coins. Know exactly how much you start with. Don't overstock the till. It is not a safe practice to have too much cash on hand. Keep the cash in a safe place, either a cash register or a cash box. You may want to keep excess cash in a safe in your office.

Designate who in your salon will be authorized to handle cash. Will each cosmetologist collect money from the customers, or will the receptionist act as cashier? However you do it, set the policy for collecting money and making change and stick to it. Limit the number of people who have access to cash.

Deposit the money in your bank account as soon as possible, at least no later than the end of the business day. Keep out only enough to make change the next day. Use cash only to make change. Anytime you disburse money in the salon, except for change or for returned merchandise, write a check. Don't give up cash unless it is necessary. The idea is for cash to come in, not go out. Remember your cash flow. Any time you disburse cash, make out a debit slip. Enter the date, the amount, the purpose, and to whom it went. Many times when paying by check or credit card, a client will include a tip for the technician. Note that amount. Give that amount to the technician in cash. Don't forget the debit slip. You will have to account for that cash later.

Be careful when handling cash. Examine the money you receive to be sure it is genuine. Counterfeiting is always a threat to a cash business. If you accept a counterfeit bill, you're stuck with it. You have to surrender it to the authorities and you will not be reimbursed for the loss.

If you get a counterfeit bill, follow the Secret Service Department guidelines. Don't return the bill to the passer. Note his or her description and the license number of any vehicle he or she uses. Call your local police or the Secret Service office. Handle the note as little as possible and put it in an envelope for protection. Surrender it only to a properly identified police officer or U. S. Secret Service agent. Cooperate fully with the authorities. The booklet, *Know Your Money*, available from the Government Printing Office, contains information on recognizing counterfeit money and what to do about it.

Handling Checks

Decide whether you will accept personal checks for payment. Many customers find it convenient to pay for services by check instead of cash, and you may want to extend that convenience to them. Be aware that there is more risk in accepting checks than in a strictly cash transaction. Bad checks are a major problem and, once accepted, are difficult to collect. In addition, you do not have use of the money until the check clears the bank. That may take anywhere from three to seven working days. If you choose to accept personal checks from your customers, establish definite policies and post them conspicuously in the salon.

Your best protection against bad checks is to know your customer. If you don't know the customer personally, make sure you get two forms of identification, such as a driver's license and a credit card or employee I.D. card. Record the identifying numbers on the back of the check. Don't accept checks for more than the amount of the services and purchases. Some clients may write a check for more than they owe and expect cash in change. This is a bad business practice for you. You aren't running a bank. Don't accept third party checks, either. Make sure the client signs the check and enters the correct date on it.

If a check bounces, call the client and ask him or her to make good on it. Don't take no for an answer. Be vigorous in your collection attempts. Under the law, you are also entitled to collect an additional fee for a returned check to defray the costs you will incur in the collection process.

Handling Credit Cards

You may want to give your clients the convenience of charging their purchases on a charge card or bank credit card. These are in wide use around the world and offer the salon the ability to offer credit without assuming the risk or the bookkeeping chores. You will pay a fee for the service, however, which will be a percentage of the sale. Generally, the higher the volume of business you do with the cards, the lower that percentage will be.

There are two types of cards in general use—charge cards and credit cards. Charge cards, such as those issued by American Express and the Diner's Club, let the user charge purchases from participating businesses. The user is obligated to pay the amount in full at the end of the payment period in which the charge appears on the bill and pays no finance charge if the bill is paid on time. Credit cards, such as MasterCard, VISA, Discover, and the American Express Optima Card, allow the customer to extend payments over a period of time by making a monthly payment that includes part of the principal and interest. This distinction is not of great concern to the business that accepts the cards.

There is a third type of card coming into vogue—the debit card. The purchaser uses the card to buy the services or merchandise, like a credit card, but the amount is deducted electronically from his or her bank account.

Apply for authorization to accept MasterCard and VISA from the bank with which you have your business account. Apply for authorization for the other cards directly with the issuing company. In either case, make sure you are familiar with their terms and regulations. Find out what percentage they will charge and how long it takes for the money to be deposited into your account once you've deposited the sales receipts. This is an important question. The faster you get the money, the better for your cash flow. Some card issuers take longer to deposit the money than others.

Know what risks you must assume with respect to fraudulently used cards and what risks the issuer assumes. Most card issuers require you to get prior authorization from them if the amount is above a certain limit. As long as you receive clearance from them, you have no risk. You'll get paid, whether or not the purchaser pays the bill.

Know the verification procedures established by the card issuer. Some issuers supply a booklet each month listing cards that have been revoked. If you have such a book, check the card number against it. If the card is listed, do not accept it. With some cards, you will also have a telephone number to call for authorization. In any case, be careful how you handle the cards. Anytime you accept a credit or charge card, verify the identity of the purchaser, authenticate the signature, note the expiration date on the card, and take note of the kind of card it is.

You will write the purchase on a multipart form supplied by the issuer, usually with the help of a credit card imprinting machine. The purchaser gets one part; you keep one; the bank or other institution gets the rest. Fill out the form carefully. Make sure the information on the card has been imprinted onto the form. In the spaces provided, enter the type of card, the date of the transaction, and the authorization number, if you have received one. List the items and services that have been purchased and their individual prices. Total up the prices plus tax, if any, and enter the amount. Make sure the arithmetic is correct and that all entries are legible. Make sure the customer signs the form. If the form has carbon paper for the copies, remove the carbons and give them to the customer.

Take care of the completed forms. Like checks, they represent cash. If they are lost, you may have no recourse to collect the money. Deposit the slips when you deposit your cash.

Handling Gift Certificates

Selling gift certificates for salon services is a good idea. Gift certificates are notes for presold services. They represent money you receive now for services you will provide later. They are an additional source of revenue for your salon, and can also be a source of new business.

Remember, however, that gift certificates are negotiable instruments and should be handled like cash. Keep blank certificates in a secure place. When you sell a gift certificate, make sure the amount is legible. Date all certificates. Keep a record of who purchased it, the certificate number, the gift amount, and the date.

Always know how many gift certificates you have outstanding. As they are cashed in, cross them off your list. Once sold, that gift certificate represents an obligation on your part. Treat it like a business debt.

Daily Reconciliation

Regardless of the form of the income—cash, check or credit card—you must reconcile your books at the end of each working day. This can be somewhat of a hassle, especially when you're tired after a busy day, but it is vital.

Collect the sales slips for the day and add up the totals. Total up the debit slips for any cash disbursed and subtract the amount from sales totals. Add up the totals for the cash on hand, the credit card slips, and checks, and subtract the amount of cash you started with in the till. The two amounts should be equal. In effect, you are matching the amount you should have with the amount you actually have. If there is a discrepancy, find out why. Check all the arithmetic. Doublecheck all the figures. Reconstruct the day as best you can to see if you can figure where any missing money went.

If all the arithmetic is correct and the figures still don't reconcile, you have either forgotten some disbursements or you may have a problem with theft. Review your record keeping procedures and security precautions. Note the amount missing, and inform your bookkeeper and accountant. Keep a closer watch over the record keeping and cash handling procedures in your salon.

When the figures are reconciled, enter the amounts into the proper journals and deposit the money in your account. Do this as soon as possible. Don't leave cash in the salon overnight.

RECORD KEEPING IN THE SALON

It is impossible to overstate the need for good record keeping in your salon. Accurate records do more than let your accountant figure out how much you owe in taxes. They are the means by which you know how successful your salon is. They tell you whether you're operating at a profit or a loss. They tell you which services are profitable and which are not, and they help you in both your short-range and long-range planning for the future. They are the scorecard by which you assess your business success. (Many of the more technical aspects of financial record keeping are covered in Chapter 9.)

Proper record keeping starts with the sale. Give each cosmetologist a supply of sales slips. Stock forms are available from stationery stores, or you can design your own and have them printed. Every transaction must be recorded on a sales slip. When a cosmetologist performs a service or sells a product, the client's name, the services or products purchased, and the prices should be itemized on the sales slip, which should be turned in with the cash. Each cosmetologist should initial the slip. These sales slips will become an integral part of your record keeping, so be thorough with them. They are your primary record of who did what, to whom, when, and for how much.

By the same token, record every cash disbursement on a debit slip. Note the amount and the reason. Keep these with the sales slips. At the end of the day, both will be part of your daily reconciliation procedure.

Don't think that records are only for financial purposes. You also need employee records (see Chapter 10), inventory and purchase records (see Chapter 11), and customer records. Establish and maintain a complete customer database. Make a file on every client who comes into your salon. The file should contain the customer's name, address, telephone number (both home and work), birthday (but not necessarily age), preferences, and any personal items that may be pertinent. Itemize all services and products the client purchases, along with the dates and any comments about the service. Also, record any comments and suggestions the customer offers. With a new client, ask why he or she left the salon patronized before. Was he or she dissatisfied with something there? If so, make sure you don't make the same mistake. Learn from other salons' experiences. Make sure all entries are legible, and keep them current.

The information contained in the customer file will enable you to do a better job of satisfying your clients. They will also give you valuable data about your services. Don't be afraid to ask the clients for the information. Every part of it is useful. The address lets you make mailings to your customer base. You might use this to send Christmas or Chanukah cards, announce specials, or mail your own newsletter. The telephone number is important so you can reach the client if there is a delay in his or her appointment. Knowing the birthday is valuable if you want to send each client a birthday card. This is a very nice, but often overlooked, touch that builds customer goodwill.

If you have some personal information about the customer, you can handle conversations better and give friendlier and more personal service. For example, if you know that the customer has children, you'll be able to inquire about their health when the client comes in. You don't have to ask specific personal questions to get this information, however. As you talk to the client, much of this information will surface. Just write it down when you learn it. Be careful not to intrude on the client's privacy or seem to pry by asking too many questions of a personal nature.

By keeping a record of the client's purchases of services, you can establish patterns in his or her patronage of your salon. This lets you make some predictions about future business, which is necessary for your long-range planning, and it helps you keep track of your repeat business. If you know the customer's pattern, you can send out reminder cards as the time for another service approaches. The information may also be a good indicator of when you are losing repeat business.

For example, suppose your records show that for the past year Mrs. Jones has come in for a facial every third week. As the time for the next facial approaches, you can remind her of it, either by sending a card or by bringing it to her attention when she next comes in. Suppose though, Mrs. Jones hasn't come in for eight weeks. This break in the pattern might tell you something. You may want to call Mrs. Jones and ask if there is a problem with your service. She may have been on vacation, been ill, or been dissatisfied with the service she received the last time she was in. You won't know, however, unless you ask. Don't worry about annoying her with the call. In all likelihood, she will appreciate your concern and the fact that you consider her patronage important. Just be careful not to overdo calling.

Each time a customer makes an appointment, pull up his or her file and review the information on it. Be ready for the client when he or she comes in. Know your clients.

The point is that unless you are aware of your customers' patterns of patronage, you'll never be aware of problems early enough to do something about them. You cannot have too much information on which to make business decisions. Get that information whenever you can.

But remember, it is not enough just to gather the information. You also have to analyze it. Take time to review the data you've collected and make inferences about your business. Look for the patterns that develop and adjust your business procedures as needed, according to what the data tells you. Pay special attention to your clients' comments and suggestions. You can learn a lot about your business by listening carefully.

Develop a system for recording and accessing the information you gather as it is no good to you if you can't find it when you need it.

Although you can do an effective, accurate job of information handling without a computer, you might want to computerize your record keeping. (This topic is covered in Chapter 14.) If you choose not to computerize, make sure your files are orderly and legible.

SUMMARY

It is important that you operate your salon properly. How well you do this affects your profitability, possibly even the survival of the business. The one most important item you must keep in mind is that you have to satisfy the customer. If you don't, nothing else will matter.

To operate your salon successfully you must perform services competently, be consistent in your operations, and be considerate of your customers and your employees.

Customer satisfaction is the key to repeat business. You must know what your customers want and then satisfy those wants to build loyalty to your salon. In the course of business, you'll come into contact with a wide variety of customers, each with specific needs and wants. You'll have to be able to work with all kinds of people. Some may be dissatisfied or angry; some may be disagreeable or disruptive. You must be able to cope with the situation.

Establish a set of salon policies. Write them down and make sure all your employees know what they are. Then follow those procedures consistently and evenly. Make sure they apply to all employees, even yourself.

The ambience of your salon is also important. Make sure it is an inviting place for the customer. The salon should be friendly, warm, and courteous as well as clean, orderly, and attractive. Your employees should maintain proper demeanor at all times, and you and they should always act in a professional manner.

Be careful how you schedule appointments. Don't get in the habit of scheduling appointments so closely that customers have to wait. Set your schedules so that the customer begins receiving the service on time. An appointment is a commitment that you should honor.

Your telephone is a valuable tool for your salon. Make sure it is used properly. Use it for business only. Employees and customers should not use the salon phone for personal calls. Consider putting in a pay phone for those uses. You may want to consider getting an 800-number service to make it easier for customers to call you.

Control the payment for your services. Decide whether you will accept only cash or will take checks or credit cards. Handle the cash carefully, and authorize only certain people to handle it. Keep track of every transaction. Be able to account for all cash at the end of the business day. When accepting checks, be careful. Know the customer. Take steps to collect on all bad checks, and don't give up on collections.

Keep adequate records. Good records let you know what is happening with your business. Start record keeping at the level of the sale. Have each employee make out a sales slip for each customer, showing all transactions and amounts. Use the information to amass a customer data base and to gather statistical information on the services you offer. Analyze the information periodically and use the data in your planning.

SALON RETAIL OPERATIONS

C H A P T E R

THIRTEEN

Retailing, selling products and accessories related to your salon services, can add good profit dollars to your bottom line. You must recognize, however, that although there are many similarities in selling services and selling products, there are also differences that you must consider. These include the different products and accessories you stock and sell, the way you display the goods, the competition you face, and a little different thinking in your approach to the business.

To be successful, your retail operation has to be more than just an afterthought. You have to manage that part of the operation with the same zeal and care that you use to manage the salon part. Make the retail operation a profit center for the salon business. Keep the two operations separate. Retail sales represent one mode of business; the services represent another. Don't blur the distinctions between the two.

Keep separate records and inventories for the two sides. As a profit center, the retail operation should earn revenues. Granted, this side of your business is to provide an additional service to customers, but that's no reason it should lose money. By keeping the sides separate, you can monitor the profitability of both operations. Otherwise, it is very easy to overlook losses from the retail end because of the inability to isolate those dollars from profits in the service end.

Above all, don't lose sight of your primary business—selling services. That is where the majority of your income comes from, not from retail sales. (If the opposite is true, you're probably in the wrong business.) Don't spend so much time and effort selling products that you shortchange the service part of the business. Give retailing the attention it deserves in your overall operation but no more.

THE MARKET FOR RETAIL SALES

The potential market for retail sales of cosmetics and nail and skin products by salons is enormous. Industry studies estimate salon sales of such products are better than one billion dollars each year, with tremendous opportunity for further growth. So the opportunities are there; it's up to you to capitalize on them.

You have a captive market for the products you sell. Your retail customers will come from the ranks of your client base. You take care of their beauty needs and have developed a good relationship with them, so they trust your experience and professional expertise. They are predisposed to buy their retail products from you as long as you can add value to the product. You have to give the clients a reason to buy products from you, rather than from another retail outlet. There's no reason why your client should buy a bottle of skin cleanser from you for $10.00 when he or she can buy a bottle of off-the-shelf skin cleanser for $3.00 from the local supermarket, unless you give her more value for her money; that is, better product, better service, more confidence.

While your market is captive, however, it is also limited. Don't expect to get significant walk-in business for retail items. It won't happen because you haven't built up a relationship with those people and they have no reason to trust your expertise. To build business for your retail operation, you first have to increase your customer base for the service operation, which should be your priority anyway.

COMPETITION IN RETAIL SALES

The competition for sales of salon items is intense. Surprisingly, though, it does not come from other salons. You are competing with them for the service business. Clients who patronize your salon for various services are not likely to go to another salon just to purchase products. If they are going to purchase products from a salon at all, they'll buy them in the same place they buy their services. Your retail sales competition comes from a variety of other sources that have little or nothing to do with the salon business, including drugstores, supermarkets, discount stores, department stores, specialty shops, and direct marketing organizations.

Drugstores and supermarkets typically sell mass market products as opposed to the professional, upscale products you would handle. They operate on the principle of high volume and low margins, making only a small amount on each sale, but earning their income on the large volume of sales they make. They offer no service or expertise. The consumer just walks down the aisle, drops the product into a shopping cart, and pays for it at the checkout counter. There is no added benefit; price alone is the key.

Discount stores, like drugstores and supermarkets, also sell mass market cosmetics products on a high-volume, low-margin basis. They are usually very low overhead, self-service operations. Some discount stores also sell upscale market products; however, in some cases, these may be gray market or counterfeit products. These stores also sell distressed merchandise, that is, products that they've purchased cheaply from another store that has gone bankrupt or discontinued merchandise from manufacturers or wholesalers. Here, also, price alone is the driving force behind sales.

Department stores usually concentrate on upscale cosmetics, especially makeup and skin care products. They provide service as well as sales, and the products are sold by trained personnel. In many cases, however, the personnel are trained only in one manufacturer's product line and do not have the broad training of licensed cosmetologists. Department stores have reasonably high volume sales of these products and get good margins. They also enjoy good marketing and promotional support from product manufacturers. The cosmetics department operations are quality oriented and price is less of a factor.

Specialty shops devote their entire efforts to cosmetics products usually from one manufacturer, although they may be sold under a private label. Some of these operations can be quite narrow in their specialization. For example, there are some shops that market only nail products, others that sell only makeup, and some that handle only skin and body care products. The specialty shops also enjoy very good marketing and promotional support from the manufacturers, who in some cases may be their parent company. These shops, like department stores, concentrate on upscale rather than mass market products. Store personnel are usually well trained and knowledgeable about the products and their proper use, and service is normally very good. Quality rather than price is the key to their success.

Direct marketing organizations include those who sell cosmetics products door-to-door, by mail through catalogs, and by infomercials on television. Door-to-door operations utilize a veritable army of salespeople who either go from house to house or set up demonstration parties in a willing customer's house and solicit orders for the products. These companies normally market upscale products at reasonable prices and usually limit their product lines to their own brand name products. The salespeople are generally better trained in selling techniques and product knowledge than in proper use of the materials. They offer some degree of service, but not at the level of a department store or specialty shop.

Catalog houses send printed catalogs and circulars to mailing lists they either amass or purchase from direct mail list brokers. They accept orders either by mail or by telephone and ship the goods to the buyer. The buyer never sees a salesperson. They usually carry a fairly broad line of upscale products, but sell by price and delivery. Service is nonexistent. Some of the door-to-door operations also sell through catalogs.

Infomercials are one of the newest direct marketing tools. These are paid television broadcasts, usually of thirty-minute duration, in a format that resembles a talk or game show. The entire program is devoted to the demonstration and sale of some product. A number of cosmetics products are being marketed this way. Once the province of cable channels and late night television, these programs have begun appearing on network affiliates during prime time. The sales pitches are geared to one specific product or line of products and sales are made by telephone and by mail. Price is often a factor, and product quality varies with the reputation of the manufacturer. Service is nonexistent.

Although there is some degree of competitiveness, you can't really consider yourself in competition with drugstores, supermarkets, and most discount stores, although you may face some limited competition from those particular discount stores who sell gray market or counterfeit professional, upscale cosmetics products. You won't be selling mass market items, or at least you shouldn't be, nor are you targeting the same customers. It would be impossible for you to attract the high volume of shoppers they get, or match them in price. Nor are you competing with catalog sellers or those who market through infomercials. These people have targeted a completely different audience than the one you can reach.

You are more in competition with department stores, specialty shops, and home sales organizations. Your customers probably already shop in the department stores and have ready access to the specialty shops. And it's very hard to match the convenience of the home sales companies. You cannot compete with these retail outlets in price. They have a tremendous advantage in their ability to purchase goods in large quantities and low prices. With the discount structures they receive they can sell products at prices lower than your purchase prices. Plus, they get a considerable advantage with the promotional and marketing assistance they receive from the manufacturers.

You do have a tremendous advantage, however, in the personal relationships you've built up with your clients. By offering a good mix of products they can't get in other locations and by selling them on your better service and expertise, you can capture your share of the market, even in this highly competitive atmosphere. Trust and knowledge add value to the products you sell.

PRODUCTS FOR RETAIL SALES

Your choice of products to sell at retail is important to the success of this end of your business. You want to stock products that will move, not sit on a shelf and get dusty. That means you have to tailor your product mix to the needs and tastes of your clientele. You have to be aware of trends in fashion, the beauty industry, and society as a whole. And you have to be ready to change your product mix as these trends and fashions change.

For example, there is a growing concern with the purchase and use of environmentally sound products. The "green marketing" revolution has concerned consumers looking for products that don't harm the environment. In the salon industry, this includes items such as the newer, low-volatile organic compound (VOC) hair sprays, which reduce the amount of volatile organic compounds released into the atmosphere. Also included is an emphasis on using recyclable or biodegradable materials for packaging, and reducing the amount of packaging used for products, as well as the manufacture, sale, and use of products that do not rely on animal testing. There is also more emphasis on the use of natural materials in products, as opposed to synthetic ingredients. Choose products that mirror these trends. Your customers will be looking for them.

Product Choices

As discussed in Chapter 11, sell the same products you use in your services. These are the products you know and can recommend, and will complement your services. Also, the fact that you use them in your operations adds credibility to their appearance on your retail shelf. If you don't use a product, you'll be hard put to convince your client to buy it.

In general, the same strictures apply to your retail products as to your operational products. Limit the number of brands you carry, and stock and sell only quality products. Try to pick products from manufacturers who support the salon business and don't sell their products over-the-counter to the general public in competition with salons. This can make your choice very difficult, since many manufacturers sell to both sides. A few do not, however.

Sell products that are relevant to your salon business and match the services you offer. For example, you might sell nail polishes, makeup, skin and body care products, as well as accessories that enhance these products. These all relate to what you do. You should not sell handbags, ladies' dresses, or men's ties unless you intend running a general store instead of a beauty salon. Remember your primary business. Don't carry anything in the retail operation that detracts from that business, either by diluting your efforts or by diminishing your professional image.

Know your products well. Know their ingredients and what they do. Be aware of the environmental aspects of their manufacture. Be able to answer your customers' questions and explain why that product is best for him or her.

Private Labeling

You can sell brand name items or you can sell private label products. Private label products are items you purchase unlabeled from a manufacturer on which you put your own name. Unless you have a large operation with an industry-wide reputation, private labeling will probably not work for you as there are a lot of disadvantages to it. You lose the advantages of brand recognition and can't take advantage of the money and efforts the manufacturer of the brand name products has spent to advertise and promote those products to the general public.

Remember the importance of image. You'll have to spend a considerable amount of money to have a competent graphic artist design a label for you, then spend more money to have those labels printed or silk-screened onto the bottle. In addition, you'll have to buy the labels in a fairly large quantity, which means you'll have to store them so they won't get dirty or damaged until you can use them. Then you have to apply the labels to the bottles or jars. You'll also have to purchase the unlabeled products in larger quantities than you would brand name products, increasing the possibilty of spoilage or passing an expiration date. And when all is said and done, and you've spent the money and done what promotion you could, you still don't have a unique product. You wind up with virtually the same products carried by all the other salons who are private labeling. The only thing different is your label. The ego trip of having your own name brand isn't worth the money or the effort it takes.

Stick with brand name products for your retail sales. Take advantage of the manufacturer's reputation and marketing and promotion efforts. Work with the known quantities.

Pricing

Pricing your retail products depends on a number of factors. How exclusive are the products? Who else is selling them at retail? If there is no other source for the products nearby, you can probably sell them at a higher price than if other salons in the area are selling them. Your prices will also depend on the image of your salon and the clientele you service. If you operate a low-cost, high-volume salon, your prices would be lower than if you operate a high-cost, exclusive salon. Your product mix would also be different.

While you should be competitive in pricing with other area salons that sell the same or similar products and cater to a clientele similar to yours, don't try to compete on price with other retail outlets. Simply put, you can't. There's no way you can match their purchasing power and volume. Your edge is in service and expertise, not in price. You should also have an advantage by selling exclusive products.

Whatever your situation, though, don't underprice your products. Charge what they're worth, and allow yourself a fair markup. You have to make a profit from the sales, so you have to charge enough to do that. You know how much the products cost you. Don't forget to add in other costs, such as shipping and handling, commissions, and a fair share of the salon overhead, when you figure out the cost of each product. The manufacturers have probably suggested retail prices for the products. These price suggestions are based on their research and on the knowledge of what prices the products will command around the country and include a reasonable markup based on industry averages. Those suggested retail prices are a good starting point. How much you will deviate from those is up to you. You may, if you choose, settle for a somewhat lower price to meet specific situations. You may also charge more, but it will take exceptional circumstances to be able to do this successfully.

RETAIL INVENTORY MANAGEMENT

You have to be just as careful managing your retail inventory as your operational supply inventory. Like any supplies, those products you stock represent cash. Don't overbuy. You don't want to tie up your capital in items that will sit on a shelf or in your storeroom for any length of time. But make sure you get what you need. You can't sell what you don't have.

This might sound contradictory, but it's part of the balancing act you have to work on. In the beginning, at least, you won't have much information and will have to make educated guesses as to what products will move and what won't. As you gain experience and keep good records, this task will become easier.

Keep your retail stock separate from your operations stock. You are operating the retail end as a profit center. If you mix retail with operational products, it will be harder to track the results. You also lose your economies of scale. Even though you should be selling the same items at retail as you use in the salon, many of your retail products will come in smaller, consumer-sized packaging as opposed to the larger, professional packaging. For example, suppose you use a name brand skin cleanser in the salon and you purchase this in one-quart bottles. For retail sales, you would purchase that same cleanser in eight-ounce bottles. The unit cost for the smaller bottles is more than for the large containers; thus, it is not economical for you to use the smaller bottles in your salon. It costs you more money and eats into your profitability.

Review the sections on determining supply requirements and quantities in Chapter 11. The principles are the same. As with other supplies, keep the retail products locked in a storeroom. Limit access to the materials and the number of individual packages of any item you have displayed for sale, and restock the shelves and counters as necessary. For example, you might stock twenty-four bottles of skin cleanser, but will display only six at a time. And, as you did with the other supplies, set up an inventory control card system so you can keep track of the items. Set minimum, maximum, and reorder quantities for each item, just as you did with the others.

Be aware of expiration dates. Many products have limited shelf life. Know which ones they are. Rotate your stock so you sell the oldest products first. If a product on display passes that date, remove it from the shelf and discard it. Manufacturers put expiration dates on products for good reason. After a certain time, they may spoil. You might sell an outdated product and it might work fine, but the risk you run, either in customer dissatisfaction or customer health, isn't worth it.

Keep meticulous records on your retail sales. Enter all sales in your log books. Know where and when each item went and for how much it sold. Gather all the data you can and analyze it regularly. Look for information that tells you which products sell best and how long it takes each product to sell. This data will help you when it comes to deciding which products to keep, which to discontinue, and what quantities of each product you should stock. Also keep records on which products you have to discard because they have become out-dated. The price data lets you figure the profitability of each product.

If a client returns a product, record that information. Ask why the product is being returned, and look for patterns. Are particular products coming back with any frequency? Are they coming back for the same reasons? Use this information in your decision making.

THE RETAIL SALES AREA

The area in which you conduct your retail sales is an important feature of your salon and should be designed with the same criteria as any other section. (See Chapter 5 for a review of those principles.) The area should be bright, clean, well lit, and as roomy as possible. If you have a separate room for retail sales, make sure it is visible from the reception area and the outside. Ideally, patrons should have to pass through the retail area on their way in or out of the salon.

Product Display

Your retail area should be inviting and attractive and should catch the awareness of the clients as they pass through it. Keep it neat and uncluttered, and arrange the products to focus attention on them. Display the products to show them to their best advantage. You can place them in glass display cases, on counter tops, in bins, on shelves, or a combination of any of these. In some cases, you might put selected products on a free-standing pedestal to call special attention to them. Keep the more valuable items in locked display cases to guard against shoplifting. Change your product display frequently to keep a fresh look in the area. If you keep the same display for a long time, your clients can become so used to it, they won't notice it.

Keep glass display cases, counter tops, and shelves clean and free of fingerprints and dust. Clean the products frequently, too. Mark the price clearly but unobtrusively on each item. Decide whether you want the customers to serve themselves or have a designated salesperson wait on them. Self-service items need to be accessible, placed on open shelves or in bins. Items in display cases will not be self-service.

The overall illumination in the retail area should be bright and even, but you can highlight certain products with spotlights. Be careful if the products are exposed to sunlight coming through your windows. The ultraviolet radiation can cause colors to fade and destroy the appearance of the products.

Use appropriate props to show off the products. For example, you might use a bed of autumn leaves to display an assortment of makeup in seasonal colors. Keep a supply of things you can use for props, such as cotton batting, assorted colors of cloth for drapings, ribbons, and mirrors. Color coordinate your displays. The displays should be harmonious, not discordant.

Always be alert for product display ideas. Visit department and specialty stores and see how they display their goods. Look at various magazines to see how products are shown in advertisements. Start a clipping file of display ideas, and use your imagination.

Take advantage of point-of-purchase displays, posters, and promotional exhibits you can get from the product manufacturers. Ask your supplier what materials are available. Use demonstrations and samples when you can get them. Also, store fixture distributors sell display accessories. Obtain a catalog and visit their showrooms to get display ideas.

RETAIL SELLING

Decide who in your salon will handle retail sales. You have a number of choices—your receptionist, your technicians, or yourself. Unless retail sales make up a major part of your business, you probably won't need or be able to afford a full-time retail sales clerk.

Whoever you choose to handle sales, however, should be fully trained in the products and able to answer any questions that arise. Include the duties in the job description for the position so there won't be any disagreements over the responsibilities. Decide on the form of compensation you will give for the job. Will it come in the form of extra pay, or will you pay a commission on each sale? If you have only one or two people making sales, extra pay might be suitable; however, if you leave the task to each cosmetologist, a commission might be better.

Success in retail sales takes some degree of salesmanship. You have to know what motivates people to buy. You must understand their needs and be able to show them how the product meets those needs. As discussed in Chapter 12, know the difference between the features of the products and their benefits. The features are the attributes of the product; the benefits are what it accomplishes for the client. Whether they realize it or not, the clients buy the benefits, not the features. They want to look and feel good. Their concern is whether the product will accomplish that; your concern is to convince them that it will.

Know both your clients and your product. You've worked on your clients' skin or nails and should know the condition they're in. You should also know how the products you sell work, especially if you're also using them in the services you sell. Be able to match the product with the customer. After all, your edge in the retail end of the business is your professional expertise. You should know what will suit the clients best. They will normally accept your judgment and rely on it.

You might hold an occasional sale, where you offer selected products at a reduced price, even a price at or below your actual cost. This is especially helpful when you are introducing a new product and want people to try it. Try to avoid loss leaders, which are products sold at an artificially low price as an inducement to get people to come into the store. This is offered with the idea that, once inside the store, the customers will purchase other items at their normal prices, as well. This kind of sales strategy will not usually work with a salon, because you're not drawing customers from outside your client base.

Many of the sales you make will be on impulse as opposed to planned. That is, the customers have not come into the salon with the intention of buying a product but for the service. They have, however, accepted your recommendation and understood how the product will benefit them. And they've made the purchasing decision. You have sold them.

You have to sell the products. They won't sell themselves. Customers usually will not buy a product from you unless you have suggested it to them and convinced them it is right. But you won't make the sale unless you ask for the order. Don't be afraid to try to sell a product to a client, but don't overdo it. Hard sells don't work; they only alienate the customers.

There's an important point in salesmanship. Once you've made the sale, stop selling. The customer has made the decision to buy. He or she doesn't need any more convincing or reinforcement. More sales are lost because the salesperson keeps talking about the product after the customer has made the decision to buy it.

Above all, be ethical in your retail sales efforts. It's just as important here as in your other salon operations. Don't sell a product just to make the sale. Make sure the product is right for the client. If you truly believe it is, don't be afraid to suggest it. Stand behind the products you sell. Offer a money back guarantee, whether or not you can return the product to your supplier. Your own personal guarantee is necessary to reinforce the customer's confidence.

SUMMARY

Retail sales are an excellent opportunity to increase the profitability of your salon. However, there are differences between selling services and selling products. You have to manage both aspects of the business equally well, but you can't let the retail sales side dominate the services side. Remember your primary business.

The potential market for retail sales of specialized salon products is large, but it is made up of your customer base. You won't be able to compete with large chain stores or department stores. You have to find your own special niche, then make your sales to the people who purchase your services.

You have a wide choice of products to offer for sale. By and large, they should be the same products you use in the services you offer. You should match the selections to the needs of your customers. You should only sell products that are relevant to your business and mirror the services. Know the products well, however, and be able to discuss their benefits and features with the clients. Price the products according to their value. Don't underprice. You can't compete on price, so don't try, but offer service with the products to increase their value.

Manage your inventory carefully. Inventory represents money. Don't overstock, but have enough product on hand to meet your needs. Keep records of all retail sales. Know which products move and which don't, and adjust your inventory accordingly.

Display the products attractively to show them to their best advantage. If possible, have a separate retail sales area. Designate one or more employees, trained in both salesmanship and product knowledge, to handle retail sales.

CHAPTER
FOURTEEN

In the modern business world, a computer has become a virtual necessity. You can conduct your business without one, but using one can make your job a lot easier. Computers can handle many tasks in the salon, from helping you manage your customer base to generating financial reports, but it is not a panacea. It is a help, a tool, not a miracle worker. It doesn't replace common sense and thought on your part. A computer doesn't think or make decisions for you. It is just a dumb machine that is only as good as the information you put into it. There is a term for this in computer circles—GIGO, which stands for Garbage In; Garbage Out. So if you use a computer in your salon, make sure you know how to use it properly.

At one time, not so long ago, computers were large and very expensive machines that were difficult to operate. Their cost and complexity made their use prohibitive in small businesses. Those times are gone. In the past few years the number of computer manufacturers has greatly increased and machines have gotten smaller and easier to use. And their cost has come way down. At the same time, many relatively low cost programs have become available to make the computer an effective tool for business. Now, a computer system is a very practical and cost effective acquisition for small businesses. Salons are no exception.

CHECKLIST 14-1
USES OF THE COMPUTER

There are many possible uses for a computer in the salon, including:

1. Maintaining customer lists
2. Keeping records of customer services
3. Scheduling and making appointments
4. Keeping employee records
5. Word processing for letters and other documents
6. Accounting and bookkeeping functions
7. Inventory control
8. Managing and analyzing business data

USES OF THE COMPUTER

The computer can handle many jobs in the salon. Its uses are limited only by your imagination. As you gain experience, you will undoubtedly find many ways to make it work for you. Most users put them to work in a variety of applications.

Customer lists. You can keep your customer list on file, with the ability to access any customer by name, address, telephone number, preferences, frequency of patronage, birthday, and personal information. This becomes your basic mailing list that lets you send special notices, holiday greetings, and birthday cards to each customer.

Customer service records. You can keep a record of customer purchases of services, with a notation when the next service is due, so you can send a reminder card to the customer. It also lets you know the results of all services performed and keep track of specific information, such as skin care products used.

Scheduling and appointments. You can establish a calendar with the computer that will let you keep track of appointments, employee schedules, and dates of trade shows and industry meetings you might attend.

Employee records. You can keep all of your employee information on file, with the ability to call up any information from attendance records to pay data.

Word processing. You can write letters and memos and generate other documents, including your Employee Handbook, Salon Procedure Manual, or even a customer newsletter. The computer lets you write the original document and make revisions easily.

Accounting and bookkeeping. You can keep all accounting records and financial data on the computer and use the information to generate financial reports for the bank when you apply for a loan. You can also generate profit and loss reports for tax purposes or for the use of your partners, if you have any. You can even use the computer to print checks, pay your bills, and pay your employees.

Inventory control. You can keep track of your salon and retail sales inventory. In addition, you can use the information to monitor the sale, use, and reordering of products.

Business data management and analysis. You can use the computer to help you compile and analyze information that lets you see how well your business is doing. This gives you the data you need to make prudent decisions about your salon.

You can do all of these tasks, plus a lot more, with a computer system. Granted, you can also do these things without a computer, but the machinery will make the job easier, faster, more accurate, and probably less expensive.

COMPUTER EQUIPMENT

A computer system consists of a combination of hardware and software. Hardware refers to the machinery; software refers to the programs, or instructions that tell the machinery what to do. To be functional, the system requires both. It also requires that both be compatible, that is, that they work together.

The computer's operating system is the hardware manufacturer's program that is built into it and organizes and manages all of the computer's internal functions and various parts. Hardware and software will be compatible only when they utilize the same operating system. As a general rule, if the operating systems are different, the machinery and programs won't be able to work together. There are a number of operating systems in general use. The two most common are the MS-DOS system and the Apple system. Attachments and software designed for one won't work on the other. This is an important consideration when you are buying your system. Make sure everything is compatible.

Computer Hardware

Hardware consists of the basic computing unit and a number of peripherals, devices that attach to the basic unit to perform certain functions. The minimum hardware required is the basic unit, a monitor, and a keyboard. You can add other peripherals as you need them. Some will be more useful in the salon than others.

THE BASIC COMPUTING UNIT   The basic computing unit is the heart of the system. It is the box that contains the central processing unit, the memory and, in most modern computers, one or more disk drives. It also has a series of connectors that allow you to plug in the peripherals and a cooling fan to keep the various electronic components from overheating. The brain of the system is the central processing unit (CPU), a microprocessor that performs all of the analytical and computational functions of the computer. The CPU is usually housed on the main logic board, a circuit board that holds the microprocessor as well as the RAM and ROM memory and other circuits that let the computer perform its many functions.

There are two types of memory—read-only memory (ROM) and random-access memory (RAM). Both types store information for later use. ROM can't be changed. You can read the data in the memory, but you can't alter it in any way. It is the memory built into the computer by the manufacturer and contains the instructions that let the computer start up when you turn it on. The contents of the read only memory stay in place even when there is no power going into the computer. RAM is the internal memory that takes the information fed into the computer from disks or input devices and stores it so it can be used. This memory is also built into the machine but can be both read and changed. When you turn the computer off, either deliberately or by accident, this memory is lost.

Computers are supplied with different amounts of random-access memory. The more application programs you intend to run, the more you will need. When you buy your system, make sure you get as much RAM as you will need to let the machine do everything you want. You can never have too much. Memory is measured in units called bytes. One byte generally represents one character, either a letter, number, or punctuation mark. Your computer's RAM will be rated in kilobytes or megabytes. One kilobyte equals 1,024 bytes. One megabyte equals 1,024 kilobytes or 1,048,576 bytes. So, if you have a machine with 4 megabytes of RAM, you can store 4,194,304 characters worth of information. This amount will handle most application programs.

Disk drives are devices for storing and accessing additional information. They let you use memory that is not built into the computer, i.e., memory other than RAM, by writing information onto or reading information from a diskette. There are two types of disk drives in common use. Fixed, or hard, disk drives contain a metal disk that is sealed permanently into the drive. These are very fast and hold a lot of information, typically ranging from 20 to 160 megabytes. Floppy drives utilize plastic diskettes to read or write information. Floppy disks hold much less information than hard disks, but have the advantage of being portable. You can transfer information from one computer to another, for example, by using a floppy disk, as long as both computers use the same operating system and the same application program. The two most commonly used sizes of floppy disks are 3-1/2 inch and 5-1/4 inch. Most newer computers have a fixed disk drive and one or more floppy disk drives built in. External drives of both types are also available as accessories.

The information is actually stored on the diskette, so it is not lost when the computer is turned off, as is the case with information in random access memory. Floppy disks are magnetic so should be stored away from magnets and telephones and should be handled carefully.

THE MONITOR   The monitor is a television set-like peripheral that displays the information contained in the computer. It is the device that lets you see what you are doing when you are working on the computer. Monitors are available in a variety of sizes and in either black and white or color.

THE KEYBOARD   The computer keyboard is the primary input device for the machine. They generally resemble typewriter keyboards and function in much the same way, although they also contain a number of specialized keys. You can type commands and information into the computer either with the letter and number keys or with various special function keys. Most keyboards also have direction keys that let you control the position of the cursor, a visual symbol that points to your location on the screen.

These are the items that must be present for you to have a functional computer system. There are other peripherals, however, that you may need, as well.

THE PRINTER   A printer is a device that produces paper copy from the information you've entered into the computer. There are a number of different kinds of computer printers that vary in the way they put ink on paper and in their various capabilities, such as speed and print quality. Dot matrix printers are the most common and the least expensive. These can print copy and some graphics and work by forming letters and other images with a series of pins that strike a ribbon, which deposits the ink on the paper. The quality of the print is adequate for many applications but is not up to letter-quality standards.

Daisy wheel printers work by striking a type bar on a ribbon, which transfers the ink to the paper—like automatic typewriters. They produce letter-quality print with copy but can't reproduce graphics. These are more expensive than dot matrix printers and are not as versatile. Daisy wheel printers are becoming obsolete as other printer technologies are getting less expensive.

Ink jet printers work much the same as dot matrix printers, except they squirt ink droplets onto the page instead of utilizing a ribbon. They can print both copy and graphics, and their print quality is better than dot matrix printers. But they are slightly more expensive. Some ink jet printers can print in different colors by using different color inks.

Laser printers offer the best quality of printing and can handle both copy and graphics. These devices work much like copy machines in that they put images on paper by electrostatically depositing a fine carbon powder onto the paper. They are more expensive than other types of printers, although their prices have been dropping dramatically. Laser printers are now on the market at prices well within the price range of most small businesses.

Choose your printer based on the quality of output you need and what you are going to use it for. In addition to print quality, look at features such as resolution, speed, and paper feed. Resolution is a measure of print quality and is measured in dots per inch (DPI). The higher the DPI, the better the quality of the print. Speed is measured in pages per minute. Check how fast the printer will turn out copy. Computers generally use either continuous form paper or single sheets. Typically, dot matrix and daisy wheel printers use continuous form paper, which must be separated into individual sheets by hand after printing. Ink jet and laser printers usually utilize single sheets of paper, which is normally less expensive than continuous form paper and is more versatile because a greater variety of paper grades and colors are available.

THE MODEM A modem is a device that lets your computer communicate with other computers by telephone. This can be useful if you are a subscriber to one of a number of business databases and get information from them, or if you are part of a chain of salons with a need to pass information from one location to another. Modems may be either internal (built into the computer) or external (attached to the computer as a separate accessory).

Modem performance is measured in units called bauds, and the devices come in various baud ratings. The higher the baud rating, the faster the modem transmits and receives information. This is important, since every time you use the device, you're paying long distance telephone rates. The faster your modem, the lower your telephone bill will be.

ALTERNATE INPUT DEVICES In addition to the keyboard, there are other devices for entering information into the computer. The most common of these is the mouse, a small, hand-held device that lets you point to specific locations on the screen and, by pressing its button, enter certain commands. Not all computers and computer programs can utilize this device. A mouse operates by rolling on a single ball that makes contact with the desk surface. A trackball is a type of inverted mouse, which operates by manipulating the ball directly.

THE VOLTAGE SPIKE PROTECTOR Computers are vulnerable to voltage surges coming through the electric power lines. If a surge occurs while you are working on the computer, you can lose valuable data. For this reason, you should connect the computer and its peripherals to the electric power source through a specially designed voltage spike protector, which will prevent damage and loss of information.

THE SCANNER A scanner is a device that translates images, i.e. photographs and drawings, into digital information that can be handled by the computer. This lets you add pictures to your documents and may be useful if you are an experienced computer user and are producing newsletters or other documents that contain pictures as well as words. Scanners are very expensive, although like other computer peripherals, their prices are coming down rapidly.

THE CD-ROM PLAYER   One of the newest peripherals for the computer is the CD-ROM player, a device that takes data from a laser disk and inputs it into the computer. The machine is similar to the CD player found in many audio systems. The laser disks hold a staggering amount of information that can be accessed very quickly. For example, one laser disk can hold the entire contents of a twenty-two-volume encyclopedia. The device gives you the ability to call up any entry in the encyclopedia virtually instantaneously. Unless you have a need for the types of information available on the laser disks, however, the device has only limited use for business purposes.

Computer Software

No matter how sophisticated your computer system may be, it can't do anything until it receives instructions. That is the function of the computer software, programs that tell the computer what to do and how to do it. To make your computer work, you will need a number of software packages, which are available from a number of sources. The most widely used business software comes as proprietary packages from a number of vendors. You don't really buy this software. Rather, you purchase a license to use it. You may not lend or give it to someone else to use. Software publishers protect their rights vigorously, so misuse of such proprietary software can lead to serious penalties.

Some software is in the public domain and its use is free. Such software is available through computer user groups and on community bulletin boards, and you will need a modem to access it. Other software is known as shareware. You get this type in much the same way as public domain software, but are obligated to pay a small fee for its use. Collection of the fee is largely on the honor system.

You will most likely use a number of proprietary software packages. The software comes on one or more disks, which you load into your computer memory. Most software packages come with instruction manuals and tutorials, subprograms that teach you how to use the program.

Choose your software on the basis of your needs. There are many variations of the most commonly used types of programs. They vary in complexity, cost, and ability to do the job efficiently. Shop carefully, and make sure the software package will work with your computer's operating system. Once you break the seal on a software package, you can't return it.

WORD PROCESSING PROGRAMS   Word processing programs let you write and edit documents. You would use this type of program to write customer letters, employee manuals, salon procedure guides, and the like.

DATA BASE MANAGEMENT PROGRAMS   Data base management programs organize and manage information. You would use this type of program to maintain your customer lists, your employee records, etc.

SPREADSHEET PROGRAMS   Spreadsheet programs are analysis tools for business. They let you enter a wide variety of data and then manipulate that data to make inferences about the possibilities you might have. They help you see what might happen if you make any of a number of decisions.

ACCOUNTING AND BOOKKEEPING PROGRAMS   A wide variety of accounting and bookkeeping programs are available that will let you do everything from keeping your basic financial, sales, and expense records to actually printing out checks.

DESKTOP PUBLISHING PROGRAMS   These programs let you publish your own brochures and documents by doing basic typesetting and design. With a desktop publishing program, you can integrate copy and graphics into one document. You would use it, for example, if you published a salon newsletter for your customers.

GRAPHICS PROGRAMS   Graphics programs let you draw pictures and illustrations for use in other programs. Depending on the sophistication of the program, you can create anything from a simple line drawing to a complicated painting.

CALENDAR PROGRAMS   These programs, which can serve as valuable time management tools, let you make up a calendar to keep track of appointments, meetings, etc.

VIRUS PROTECTION PROGRAMS   A computer virus is a destructive program introduced into a computer as a prank or with malicious intent. Virus protection programs seek out these viruses in your computer and erase them before they can do any damage. If you utilize only proprietary software, you may not need one of these programs. If you transfer disks from one machine to another, or get information through a modem, you should definitely have one. Their cost is minimal, compared with the cost of replacing data or programs, so it is probably a good idea to protect your computer, no matter how you obtain the data you input.

SPECIALIZED SOFTWARE PACKAGES   Some manufacturers supply software packages designed to meet most business needs. Some offer programs and equipment especially for salons.

CHOOSING YOUR COMPUTER SYSTEM AND SOFTWARE

When it comes to buying your system and software, you have a lot to choose from. Do it carefully. Take the time to think about your needs. Talk to other business computer users, and get advice from your accountant and your other advisors. Read as much as you can. Many books and magazines are available on the subject. Talk to computer salespeople. And don't believe everything anybody tells you. Find out for yourself.

Also remember, you don't need to get everything at one time. Start with the basic components and software and learn how to use them to their fullest. Then add to them as you need to.

The most important aspect is to know exactly what you want the computer to do for you. Research your needs and have a good idea of your expectations; then start looking at equipment and software. Consider your software needs first. After all, that is what does the work. Then build your computer system around the software packages. Make sure all the components are compatible.

Once you've decided, shop for the best package you can get. Don't consider price only, however. Service is very important. Look for a computer vendor who is knowledgeable, who is willing to work with you, and who provides service. Deal with vendors who are experienced in working with small business computer systems and who understand the needs of small businesses. Don't rely on verbal promises about the capabilities of any system or software. Get it in writing.

USING YOUR COMPUTER PROPERLY

Once you have your computer, take the time to learn to use it properly. Read the instruction manuals, and take the tutorial subprograms that come as part of most software packages. Many schools offer courses in computer use. Consider taking one or more. The more proficient you become, the more valuable the computer will be for you.

Consider who will use the computer in your salon and limit access to it. You don't want everybody to work on the machine. That only increases the possibility of damage and misuse. Assign the job only to those with some reason to have access to the data. The receptionist or bookkeeper, for example, might be your computer operator. Make sure everyone who is authorized to use the computer is fully trained in its use, even if it means sending them to classes.

The location of your computer is also important. Carefully consider where you will put it. The most logical place to put it is where it will be used most, probably on or next to the reception desk. Make sure the location has adequate ventilation and does not get too hot. Keep liquids away from the unit. The printer does not have to be next to the computer. Some printers can be quite noisy. Put the printer where it is convenient, but won't interfere with the operations of the salon.

You may also want to put another computer in your office. You can link the two together to use common information and a common printer. With one terminal in the office, you can work on confidential data there, while the receptionist or other employee works on the day-to-day information at the reception desk.

Security is also an important consideration. Your data is valuable. Safeguard it. Keep disks locked when not in use and secure them at night when the salon is closed. Utilize passwords, secret words that allow only those who know them to have access to the information, to limit access to the data.

Choose passwords with care. Don't use easy-to-guess words, such as your spouse's name. Change your passwords on a regular basis, and make sure you remember what they are. Otherwise you won't have access to your data either.

Enter data carefully. Make sure it is accurately put into the computer. As you enter data, save it often. Remember the discussion on RAM earlier. RAM is lost when the computer is off. If you have a power failure while you are entering data, anything you have not saved to the disk will be lost. So get into the habit of saving the data every few minutes. Once the data is on a disk, you don't have to worry about saving it. Also back up your disks frequently, at least on a daily basis. Backing up just means making copies of your disks, so you have duplicates in case of emergency.

SUMMARY

A computer is a virtual necessity in running a business. It can handle a lot of jobs in your salon and make record keeping and analysis easier.

The computer system consists of hardware (the equipment) and software (the programs that do the work). Both are important. The software must have the same operating system as the hardware. At a minimum, you need the basic computing unit, a keyboard, and a monitor, plus a printer for producing hard copy. There are many other peripheral pieces of equipment, although you can get these as you need them.

A lot of computer equipment is on the market at quite attractive prices. Before choosing one, however, do your homework. Know what you want to do with it. Be sure of your needs and expectations first, then go shopping. Make sure the computer you buy meets your needs. Then learn how to use it properly.

MARKETING, ADVERTISING, AND PROMOTION

C H A P T E R

FIFTEEN

"Build a better mousetrap and the world will beat a path to your door." There are few old sayings that are less true, especially for a business. You may offer the best services and the best values in the world, but if no one knows about them, you won't have any business. No matter how good your services may be, you'll have to market them if you expect to draw customers to your establishment.

All businesses, whether large or small, must market their services and products to be successful. Why is marketing essential to your salon? It is essential simply because consumers have a choice about where they will purchase their goods. As long as they have a choice, marketing will drive business. Remember, people don't buy things; they buy solutions to their problems. Marketing, along with marketing communications, tells them what those solutions are and helps them make the right choice.

In its most simple terms, marketing means nothing more than creating a demand for your services—making people want to come to your salon and buy what you have to offer. The term covers all of the functions you employ to get your services and products to the consumer from choosing the services you will sell, identifying the people you'll sell them to, and making the products and services attractive to the target audience, making those people aware of your services and products, convincing them to come into your salon, and making sure they are satisfied and willing to come back again.

It sounds like a tall order, and it is. But it's what you've been doing all along, whether you realize it or not. You started the marketing process when you began to develop your business plan. You continued it as you made decisions about the services and products you would offer and gathered information about your potential customers, then utilized that demographic data plus analyses of all internal and external factors that would affect your salon to make forecasts about the share of the potential market you could capture. Now you must consider how you're going to reach those potential customers, convince them to try your salon, and turn them into clients. That requires you to develop your marketing communications plan, which includes your advertising and promotional efforts. Advertising and promotion are key parts of your overall marketing strategy.

THE MARKETING COMMUNICATIONS PLAN

Your marketing communications plan is the blueprint that helps you reach your marketing goals. It helps you take your information, analyze it, and develop strategies and tactics that you will use to capture your share of the business.

Marketing Information

The marketing communications plan, just like any business plans you make, relies on information. The more you know about the situation, the better your plan will be. Information starts with your target audience. Know your audience. There is no more fundamental precept. You'll hear this time and time again.

Your demographic data form the principal base for your decision making. The accuracy of this information is crucial to your planning. (Review the sections on gathering demographic data in Chapter 2.) Who are the people you want to reach? What are their characteristics? How many of them are there in the area you will cover? What activities do they take part in? What do they like to do? Where do they shop? You should have gathered most of this information when you formulated your business plan. Here's one place you'll use it.

In addition to knowledge of your target audience, you also have to know the competitive situation. How many other salons are in the area? What services do they offer? What prices do they charge?

Which are trying to reach the same audience you are? What are their positive features? What are their negatives? You should also have this information from your business plan.

Also analyze your internal situation. What are your strengths and weaknesses? What do you offer that is unique? How good are your services? What advantages do you have in terms of what you offer, your skill, and your location? Why should anyone patronize your salon? What will customers gain from your salon that they won't get elsewhere? Be honest with yourself. This information is important to your planning.

The marketing information you gather helps you understand the composition of the market and make a reasonable forecast of its size. This forecast lets you set sales objectives; that is, determine how much of the available business you are likely to get and establish a goal (the percentage of the available business you are trying to get). Your objectives, coupled with the analyses of the competitive situation and the internal factors, help you formulate your overall marketing plan. Your marketing communications plan is part of that.

Elements of the Marketing Communications Plan

There are five essential elements to a good marketing communications plan objectives, message and positioning strategies, specific tactics, measurement procedures, and budget. The objectives are a statement of what the communication should accomplish in a specific period of time. These should be quantifiable and measurable. That is, the result must reach a specific amount and there must be some means of measuring the result. For example, a quantifiable, measurable objective might be to increase the awareness of the salon in the neighborhood from 0 percent to 20 percent in the first year of operation.

The strategy describes how you will attain the objective. Here, you determine the theme of your message to the audience and the position of your salon in the marketplace. For example, your strategy might be to use advertisements and publicity items to tell members of the target audience that your salon uses the latest state-of-the-art technology to provide a complete range of skin, body, and nail services that are guaranteed to please.

The tactics are the specific actions you need to take to make the strategy work. They should spell out what the actions will be and when they'll take place. For example, your tactics might include the preparation of a series of three advertisements that will run in one

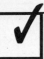

CHECKLIST 15-1
MARKETING COMMUNICATIONS PLAN

1. Marketing information
   A. Demographic data
   B. Competitive situation
   C. Salon strengths and weaknesses
2. Objectives
   A. Quantifiable
   B. Measurable
3. Strategy
   A. Message theme
   B. Positioning
4. Tactics
   A. What actions taken
   B. When taken
5. Measurement
   A. Measurement criteria
6. Budget
   A. Money allocated

local daily newspaper and one local weekly shoppers' guide on a rotating basis each week for the next thirteen weeks. Each ad will highlight one specific service—one for skin care services, one for hair removal services, and one for nail services. In addition, two publicity releases announcing new services will be sent to the local newspapers.

Measurement procedures specify how you will measure the results of the plan. The most typical way is to measure the increase in business, either by the increase in telephone calls to the salon or by walk-in trade. There should be some mechanism to determine why the new people came in. Make it a point to ask which ad or publicity notice they are responding to.

The last element, but certainly not the least important, is the budget. Determine how much it will cost to accomplish your objectives and decide how much you want to spend. Advertising and promotion represent a significant expense to the salon. Calculate your costs carefully and allocate money to the programs. Done properly, it is money well spent as it will bring in new business and increased revenues.

ADVERTISING—AN OVERVIEW

An advertisement is a paid public notice designed to call attention to a product or service with the intent of persuading the people it reaches to form a favorable opinion of the item and to purchase and use it. It can take many forms and accomplish many things. Advertising is the process you employ to develop and use the advertisements. It is both an art and a science. It can be considered a science, although an inexact one, because it utilizes scientific principles of communication and psychology. It can be considered an art, because it requires creativity and imagination to do successfully. Advertising is a means of communication, a marketing and selling tool, and a means of persuasion.

To be effective, advertising must perform three tasks. It must attract, inform, and entice. Advertising can't work if no one sees or hears it, so the first task of an advertisement is to capture the prospects' attention and interest, to make them stop and pay attention to the message. This is not an easy job in today's high-volume, media-rich environment, which bombards people with countless messages of all types. The second task is to inform the prospects about the benefits and features of the product or service, to give them the necessary data to make a decision to either purchase the goods or ask for more information. The third task is to entice the prospects, to persuade them that they need and want the product or service, and invite them to take the next step and purchase the goods.

Advertising does many things for your salon. It creates awareness of your services among your target audience by letting those people know you exist. Awareness is the first step toward purchase. No one will patronize your salon if they don't know you're there. Advertising also establishes an image for your salon among your target audience. It tells those prospects that you are a quality salon and are worth their patronage. Advertising creates a demand for your services among your target audience. Once those prospects know you exist, advertising tells them why they should patronize your salon. Advertising changes the attitudes and buying habits of your target audience. It woos the prospects away from their current salon and brings them to you. And advertising reinforces the buying habits of that part of your target audience whose business you've captured. It tells them that they've made the right choice and keeps them coming back to you.

THE ADVERTISING MESSAGE

What you say is just as important as where you say it. While it is vital to pick the right media to most effectively reach your target audience, it is equally vital to make sure they get the information you want them to get. The media and the message work together to accomplish your goals—to raise awareness of your salon and to bring in business.

Your message must lead the prospective clients to make the decision to patronize your salon. As discussed, the message must entice the prospects, inform them about your services, and persuade them to spend their money with you.

First, you have to catch their interest, so they'll read or listen to your ad. This is difficult. People are subjected to oceans of advertising every day. Commercial messages of one kind or another bombard them constantly. Test it for yourself. Pay close attention next time you listen to the radio or watch television, and count how many commercials you hear or see in one hour of programming. Note how many commercials are bundled together. To a great extent, people tune out advertising. Your ad has to stand out so it cuts through the clutter and impinges on the mind of the recipient. Then, you have to tell them what you want them to know, in terms that are meaningful to them. Finally, you have to give them good, solid reasons why they should come to you instead of to your competition.

The advertising message must be oriented to the needs of your prospective customers and should stress the benefits of your services. When people read or listen to an ad, their primary thought is, "What's in it for me?" They don't care if your salon is the biggest, the best, the most modern, if you've won every imaginable award in the beauty industry, or if your staff is world famous. Those kinds of claims in your advertising are meaningless, although you may mention some of them later in your message if, and only if, they will add credibility to your benefit statements. Don't put anything in your advertising message that doesn't work toward the goal you have set. Leave out all superfluous matter.

Positioning is an important advertising concept. This just means establishing your place in the minds of your prospects. You have to decide how you want them to think of you. What image do you want to project? What idea do you want them to have of your salon? Then, all your advertising efforts should try to build that image in your customers' minds. To do this, you must have a clear idea of who your audience is and who you are.

The principles for developing your message are essentially the same for all advertising, whether visual (print media), aural (radio), or both (television). The message has three parts—the opening, the body, and the close. The opening, or headline, has the task of capturing the prospect's attention, and should contain a strong benefit statement. It must tell the reader or listener what he or she will gain and invite him or her into the rest of the message.

Don't begin your ad with your salon name. There's no benefit in your name. That information comes later. The benefit should be specific. For example, you might open with a headline like, "Get better looking, healthier skin in thirty days." Don't ask any question that can be answered "no," as for example, "Are you unhappy with your skin condition?" If the prospect answers "yes," you have a chance, but if the answer's "no," you've lost him or her. Don't mention price in the headline. Don't, for example, say, "European-style facials, now only $35.00." You haven't yet established whether what you're offering is worth the money. At this stage, there's no perceived benefit.

The body of the message should contain proof statements for the major benefit in your headline. You've told the prospect what he or she will gain. Now you have to explain how. For example, to continue with the above sample, you might say, "A series of European-style facials given by our professional staff of estheticians will cleanse and condition your skin. Your skin will be healthier and radiant looking. We use the most modern skin care techniques and the finest products, specially for-mulated for your skin type." You can also put in additional benefit and proof statements, if you have the room. Here is where you put in your salon name, address, and other relevant information.

In the close, you ask for the sale. Make the offer. Tell the prospect what you want him or her to do. You have to do this. People won't respond unless you lead them to do it. If you are going to discuss price at all, here is where you do it. For example, the close for the skin care ad might be, "Come in for a free consultation and analysis. Call today for an appointment." You might also add a special offer, such as "This week only, get a facial for just $30.00." If you have a coupon, call atten-tion to it by saying, "With the coupon, get a facial for just $30.00."

With print ads, use illustrations, either photographs or drawings, to add visual interest to the advertisement. The illustration should support your benefit statement, if possible. A photograph of a woman receiving a facial would be suitable, but a photograph of the outside of your salon would not be so useful. You might want to utilize an equipment or product manufacturer's logo in your ad, if the manufacturer is well known. The use of such a logo can add credibility to your salon. (Of course, you should be using that equipment or product in your salon.) Make sure you get the manufacturer's permission to use the logo, as logos are protected by copyright and trademark laws. Don't overdo the use of illustrations. They should support your copy, not interfere with the message.

With radio commercials, background music and sound effects perform many of the same functions as illustrations in print advertising. They add aural interest. Here, too, don't overdo them and don't let them interfere with the sense of the message.

Obviously, the amount of information you can put in your advertising message will depend on the size of the space or length of time you buy. The larger the ad, the more you can say. However, regardless of the size of the ad, don't try to say too much. Limit your message to one major benefit, with its proof statements, plus the offer and your salon name, address, and telephone number. If the ad is fairly large, you may consider a second benefit statement, but don't clutter the advertisement up with more than that. Too much information will turn off the prospect and negate your chance for making the sale.

Be absolutely truthful in your advertising. Don't exaggerate your claims or promise anything you can't deliver. For example, you should not claim to be able to remove wrinkles permanently, unless of course, you can. Be very careful not to make any statements that could be considered medical in nature. You are operating a salon, not a hospital. You are not licensed to practice medicine, so don't claim to heal or cure anything. Stress the beauty and health aspects of your services. Be wary of comparative advertising. Don't denigrate other salons. Talk about your positive features, not their negative ones. Be as ethical in your advertising as you are in the conduct of your business.

MEASURING ADVERTISING EFFECTIVENESS

It is very important that you know how effective your advertising is. If you want to make the most effective use of your advertising dollars, you have to be able to measure the results. Make sure you have some means of doing that.

There are many different ways of measuring advertising effectiveness. The media salespeople will probably talk to you about your cost per exposure, or how much it costs to reach each member of the audience they service. For example, suppose you advertise in the local neighborhood weekly newspaper that has a circulation of ten thousand people. Your advertisement cost $300.00; therefore, your cost per exposure (cpe) is three cents. The cpe figure can be valuable when you're comparing one advertising vehicle with another, so you can make an intelligent buying decision. For example, if newspaper A has a cpe of three cents and newspaper B has a cpe of five cents, A may be the better ad buy, as long as the demographics of the audience they reach are comparable.

Unfortunately, these figures don't always tell you the whole story. To get the true picture of your cost, you need to know how many of the people the vehicle reaches are actually in your target audience. For example, even though the newspaper has a circulation of ten thousand, how many of those people are potential customers? You have to analyze the newspaper's circulation data to get that information. They will, or should, have this data. Ask to see audited figures. Demographic data are audited by independent agencies, who, in effect, warrant that the data are true and accurate. Be wary of any advertising medium that won't give you audited circulation numbers. To continue with the example, suppose that the newspaper's demographic data show that of the ten thousand people, twelve hundred match your audience demographic profile. (Remember, you won't know this unless you know the audience you want to reach.) That makes your effective cpe twenty-five cents, as opposed to three cents. When you compare one medium against another, you need to use that effective cpe figure, not the overall cpe number. It may change your decision.

The most important measure of advertising effectiveness, however, is how many people responded to each ad, and how many of those people you were able to convert into customers. That is the true test of cost effectiveness. For example, suppose of the twelve hundred potential customers reached by the newspaper, eighty people called for more information. That brings the cost per inquiry (cpi) to $3.75. The advertisement has given you eighty new names for your mailing list. That is, you now have eighty more people you can reach with telephone solicitations or direct mail advertising, whether or not you have converted them into customers as a result of the advertisement.

Now suppose twelve of those people actually make an appointment and get a facial. That one advertisement cost you $25.00 for each new customer. Granted, by the time you factor in all the costs of giving one facial, the money each person pays for that one facial does not give you any profit. In fact, you probably have lost money on that facial. The ad did what it was supposed to do, however. It brought in new business. It is up to you to keep those people as customers, so they will keep coming back and earning profits for you. The advertising won't perform that function.

To get the best value for your advertising dollars, you have to know how much business each ad brought in. That means you have to know which advertisement each new customer responded to. If you have a coupon in the ad, put a code on the coupon that tells you where it came from. Have some code in each advertisement that lets you know the source of the business. If someone calls for an appointment or for more information, make sure the receptionist or whoever answers the telephone asks the person which advertisement they are responding to.

Analyze that information. See which advertisements and which media are doing the most effective job for you. Then eliminate the ones that are not effective and concentrate your funds on those that are.

SETTING AN ADVERTISING BUDGET

Advertising is an expenditure, and is treated as an overhead expense. Just as you do with supplies, equipment, and other expenses, you must budget for your advertising efforts. You must allocate money to buy the advertising you need, both for its production and its placement in various media. Don't forget there are two parts to the process. First you have to develop and produce the ad, whether it be print, broadcast, or other media, then you have to run it.

You have to decide how much of your resources you should allocate to your advertising. Usually, you do this as a percentage of your sales. Most businesses allow 1 to 3 percent. You will probably need to spend more than that, especially if you are just starting your salon. The actual amount you spend will be determined, in part, by your goals and by the media you choose.

By now, you should know the audience you want to reach and what you want to accomplish with your advertising. You should then gather data about the various media you feel will reach your audience. Talk to the media representatives. Figure out your effective cost per exposure for each medium. Let the media representatives give you all the cost and demographic data you need to make your decision. Then choose the media that best serve your needs. In most cases, you'll want to use a mix of media, for example, a combination of telephone directory advertising and newspaper advertising as a minimum, with perhaps some direct mail and circulars.

You don't have to do all of your advertising at once. Start with a modest program, perhaps just in one or two media, evaluate the results, and expand the program as necessary. Remember frequency, though. The more times you can run an advertisement, the more people it will reach and the more they will remember it. You may be better served, at least in the beginning, by trading size for frequency. Run smaller ads, but run them more often. Also, take advantage of any cooperative advertising allowances you can get from your suppliers. These are funds given to you by manufacturers or suppliers to use for advertising, as long as you use their brand names in the advertisements.

Evaluate your advertising results constantly. Make sure you know what is working and what isn't. Don't be afraid to change either your media or your message if you aren't satisfied with the results. But, make sure you give the advertising a fair chance to work before you make the changes.

FINDING AN ADVERTISING AGENCY

Advertising can be complicated. To do it right requires knowledge of communications, of media, and of psychology. Although it is possible to do your own advertising, it is a task best left to the experts. Just as you utilize the services of attorneys, accountants, insurance agents, building contractors, and other professionals, and rely on their aid and advice, so should you utilize the services of advertising professionals. Although you will pay for their services, just as you pay for the services of the other people you hire, you'll save money in the long run. Unless you're an expert, don't make the mistake of thinking you can do your own advertising.

Look for a small, local agency that has experience in working with small businesses. Stay away from the large agencies that handle major corporations. If they accept your business at all, which is doubtful, they won't give it much attention. Get recommendations from other small businesses in the area. When you find likely candidates, interview them and review their portfolios to see what kind of work they've done. More importantly, find out the results of the advertising campaigns they've run for other businesses.

Advertising agencies typically work on a fee plus commission basis. You pay for time and materials at a fixed rate, and the agency gets a commission from the media in which they place the advertising. Cooperate with your agency. Give them the information they need to develop effective advertising campaigns and listen to their suggestions.

If there is no suitable agency available, you might be able to utilize the services of freelancers. Again, ask other business owners in the area for recommendations. Contact your local colleges and universities. Some of their teachers or students in the communications field may do freelance work.

In addition, you can often get advertising help from your local media. If you are advertising in the local newspaper, for example, staff members will usually help you write the advertisement and give you assistance in measuring the results.

ADVERTISING MEDIA

Advertising takes many forms, utilizing a number of different media designed to attain different goals, depending on the composition and location of the target audience, the ability to reach certain audiences, and cost. For your salon business, some types are more useful and cost effective than others.

No one medium will accomplish everything you want. You will have to advertise in a number of media to get the most effective reach and results. That includes print and broadcast media, direct advertising, publicity, and aggressive sales promotion. You need to utilize a good mix of advertising, but keep your message consistent in all the media you use. Make sure the message is user oriented. That is, make sure it appeals to your audience and meets their needs and desires. Sell the benefits, not the features of your services.

Word-of-Mouth Advertising

In many ways, word-of-mouth advertising is the most effective form of advertising, especially for a service business such as a beauty salon. It has a credibility no other form can match. It is the least expensive form of advertising because it is unpaid, but it must be earned. Word-of-mouth advertising depends on your reputation, and you can't buy that. You have to offer quality services and good value for the customers' money to get the loyalty that will make your clients want to tell others about you. You also have to make sure they're satisfied, so they tell others how good you are, not how bad you are.

Cultivate word-of-mouth advertising. Encourage your clients to tell their friends and neighbors about your salon. You may even offer some inducement. For example, give clients a free manicure for every new customer they bring into the salon. Just don't try to buy their recommendations. It won't work, and you might offend your customers.

Media Advertising

Media advertising includes both print and broadcast advertising, which is aimed typically at relatively large, diverse audiences, and offers a more scattered, less focused approach to prospects.

PRINT MEDIA Newspapers. These publications are devoted to disseminating items of news and also carry opinion pieces, features, and advertising. Newspapers are generally printed on inexpensive newsprint paper stock and are meant to be discarded after reading. There are many kinds of newspapers, ranging from large city daily papers to small rural weeklies, and including shoppers' circulars and limited circulation neighborhood newspapers.

For the salon, newspaper advertising can be very useful as it is relatively inexpensive and is cost effective. The advertising rate depends on the number of readers the newspaper reaches, whether they match your target audience or not. The larger the newspaper, the more expensive it will be to advertise in it, so a local weekly will usually be less expensive than a metropolitan daily. There will also be less waste because the local paper will reach more of your target audience than the paper with a wider circulation. Know your target audience. Choose the newspapers that they read and that service the area you wish to cover.

Cost is also based on the space you utilize, usually measured in column-inches—that is, how many columns wide by the number of inches high. The larger the ad, the more it will cost. Make sure your ad is large enough to do the job you intend it to do. Remember, it has to attract, inform, and entice, so don't try to save money by squeezing the message into a space too small to hold it effectively.

The third cost factor is the frequency with which you repeat the advertisement. Advertising effectiveness depends on frequency. You have to run the ad enough times to make sure that enough people see it and remember it. The more times people see an ad, the more likely they are to remember it.

You can place either display ads or classified ads in the newspaper. Display ads are larger, cover a greater amount of space, and may contain some kind of illustration. They may be placed anywhere in the newspaper. This type of ad attracts more attention and conveys more information. Classified ads are smaller, usually single-column width in special classified advertising sections, and are usually devoted to a single purpose. Help Wanted ads soliciting new employees are typical. They are contained in the Help Wanted section along with many other ads of the same type.

Classified ads are usually less expensive than display ads, but are not as effective for attracting new business. People see your display ad when they are reading the paper, and the ad catches their eye. They only see your classified ad if they are looking specifically for the item you're advertising.

Magazines. These periodicals are devoted to a wide range of special or general interests. Magazines cover almost any subject, from hobbies to home improvements to current events. Most are published on a monthly basis, although there are some weeklies, bi-monthlies, and quarterlies. They are printed on better paper stock than newspapers and are meant to have a longer life span, although most are discarded after being read. Unlike newspapers, which aim for a wide audience, magazine audiences are more specialized, although they can be quite large. Newspapers tend to be local. Their audience resides in a specific city or neighborhood. Magazines, on the other hand, tend to reach national or international audiences.

Magazine advertising is not usually a good buy for a salon because it is very expensive and the audience is usually so spread out, there is a considerable amount of waste. Advertising rates in these periodicals are based on circulation. The more people who read the magazine, the more expensive it is. Advertising is typically in the form of display ads, which are sold in page size increments. Thus, you can buy a magazine display ad that is 1/8 page, 1/4 page, 1/2 page, 3/4 page, full-page, or multiple pages. In most magazines, you can also have either color ads or black-and-white ads. Color costs more than black and white. Some magazines also offer classified advertising, usually in special sections at the back of the book. These are less expensive than display ads and serve much the same purpose as they do in newspapers.

Although magazine advertising is usually not effective for a salon, there may be an exception in local city magazines. These periodicals are devoted to a much more narrow, and usually upscale, audience and feature articles about life in the specific city they service. While ads in this kind of magazine will be very expensive, it may be worth the cost if you are running the kind of operation whose image would benefit from exposure in the journal.

Telephone Directory Advertising. Telephone directories are a form of print media, but the advertising they carry serves a somewhat different purpose. In most forms of advertising, the object is to attract, inform, and entice. The persons who see the ad are not necessarily looking for a particular item or service, so the advertisement has to pique their interest and get them thinking about it. Telephone directory advertising, on the other hand, serves those people who have already decided what they want. The purpose of the advertisement in this vehicle is to tell them where they can get it. Thus, people use the telephone directory when they are ready to make the purchase and are looking for a source.

People really use their telephone directories. According to statistics published by the Yellow Pages Publishers Association, directories reach 98 percent of households in the United States and are consulted on an average of twice a week per person. Beauty salons are tenth on the list of most-referred-to product and service categories, and draw more than 300 million references annually. Sixty percent of the people who use their telephone directory make an immediate purchase and almost 90 percent at least call the business. So, advertising in this medium can be effective.

Advertising in your local telephone directory is practically a necessity for any business. You receive a free listing in the White Pages of the directory as a result of having the telephone service. However, this consists merely of a one-line entry that lists your salon name, address, and telephone number. It provides no information beyond that. To get a listing in the Yellow Pages section, you have to purchase the space. You should consider purchasing more than the minimum listing as it can be well worth the cost for its potential to bring in new business.

Advertising in the telephone directory can take a number of forms, depending on how much you want to spend. Like other print media, you pay for the space you use in the directory and pay a monthly fee based on the size for the one-year contract term. The basic rates are determined by the size of the audience the particular directory services. Remember, directory ads run for a one-year period. Once you sign the contract, you are obligated to pay for the full year, even if you change your mind or go out of business.

In the directory, you can opt for display ads from a full page down to 1/8 page in size. Some directories also allow the use of additional colors of type and other options such as business cards, which are smaller ads in alphabetical order that give some information about the business (or you can purchase extra lines with your regular entry to provide additional information). Or you can have your salon name set in boldface type. The least expensive ad is a plain listing of your salon. You also have a choice of headings under which the ads will appear. You should advertise under all the headings that cover the services you offer, although they don't have to be all of the same size or complexity. So, if you operate a full service salon, you might consider using your largest display ad under the major heading, Beauty Salons, and smaller display ads or expanded listings under other headings, such as Make-Up and Beauty Consultants, Manicuring, and Skin Care.

Regardless of which headings you are advertising under, keep in mind that your ad will compete for attention with all of the other ads under that heading. So, it must stand out from the others. Make the ad as large as you can afford and easy to read. Keep the layout simple and uncluttered. If possible, use some kind of illustration or another color of ink, such as red, blue, or green, if that option is available in the particular directory you choose.

Give the readers all the information they need to choose your salon. Your ad should contain your salon name, address, and telephone number and list the services you offer and your hours of operation. If you can get permission from one of the manufacturers of the products you use, add their logo to your ad. Finally, add some information that tells the prospective customer why your salon is different from the others.

It is extremely important, especially with telephone directory ads, that you carefully proofread the copy and check the layout. Make sure there are no mistakes before you approve the ad, for once it is printed, you have to live with any mistakes for an entire year.

BROADCAST MEDIA   Radio. Radio is an almost constant companion for many people. Whether at home, in the car, or at work, a radio is playing somewhere. They are inexpensive and highly portable, and are used regularly. A wide variety of stations, both AM and FM, are programmed to reach specific audiences. So, for example, you can find a station that is programmed for adults from twenty-five to fifty-four years of age that plays Solid Gold music. Or you can find a station that services affluent adults and plays only classical music. In addition, there are many radio stations that cater to ethnic audiences.

You can find a radio station that reaches virtually any demographic segment of the population you want. This ability to target a specific audience, plus relatively low cost, make advertising on local radio stations a potentially effective buy for a beauty salon. But you must know your demographics, and you must tailor your message to appeal to your target audience.

Radio advertising rates are based on the reach of the station (how many people listen to it), on the time of day, or day-part, that the ad runs, and on the length of the ad, usually either thirty seconds or one minute. Day-parts are important, because people's listening habits vary widely from one time of day to another, which makes some air time more valuable than others. For example, since many people listen to the radio when they are driving to or from work, the drive time segments from Monday through Saturday are usually the most expensive. These typically run from 5:30 to 10:00 A.M. and from 3:00 to 8:00 P.M. Next most expensive time slots are normally the Monday through Saturday late morning through early afternoon, from 10:00 A.M. to 3:00 P.M. The 8:00 P.M. through 1:00 A.M. time slot is less expensive, and the least expensive time runs from 1:00 A.M. to 5:30 A.M. Sunday time slots are generally less expensive than comparable time during the week.

The larger the audience the station reaches, the more it charges for running the ads. So, you would expect to pay more for an ad on a major metropolitan radio station than you would on a small suburban radio station. Likewise, you'll pay more for a one-minute spot than you would for a thirty-second spot, although the difference will be less than twice as much. As with advertising on any medium, frequency is important. You have to air the commercial enough times to ensure that people will hear it and will remember it. Typically, you will purchase radio advertising in units called "flights;" that is, the ad will run for a certain number of times each week during the day-parts you chose for a specific number of weeks. It may rest for a number of weeks, then pick up and run again.

As with your print ads, design your radio ads carefully to attract the attention of your listening audience and give them information they need to make a purchasing decision. Open the spot with a benefit statement to get their attention, and follow it with a proof. Make sure you include the name, location, and telephone number of the salon. Put enough information in a commercial to get the job done, but don't overload the time. Have a professional announcer do the talking. Unless you are a trained speaker, don't try to do it yourself. The results may satisfy your ego, but they won't sell your services.

When you listen to the radio, pay attention to the commercials. Note what attracts you and what doesn't. Listen to how other businesses advertise. Get ideas from them, and utilize those ideas in your own radio advertising.

Television. Television has become the most powerful communications medium in the world. It has tremendous reach and influence, and it has the advantage of combining both sound and sight to transmit messages to watchers. It is also an extremely compelling, wide-reaching, and effective advertising medium, but it can be very expensive.

Broadcast television utilizes the VHF and UHF channels and is transmitted over the airwaves and received free of charge on television sets with the proper antenna systems. There are four major nationwide networks—ABC, NBC, CBS, and FOX-TV—with their local affiliate stations, in addition to local UHF stations and Public Broadcasting Service (PBS) stations. PBS is a noncommercial broadcasting service, with programming and operation costs paid for by a combination of government funding, corporate sponsorship, and private donations, and does not accept advertising.

The commercial television stations, however, earn their money through advertising revenues. Like radio, rates are based on the size of the audience they reach and, to a somewhat lesser extent than radio, on the time of day the commercial airs. Top-rated programs command the highest advertising rates, and competition among advertisers for certain time spots can be keen, which is why ratings are so important to the stations. The higher a program is rated, i.e., the more people who watch it, the more money they can charge for advertising on that program. The costs can reach astronomical proportions. For example, a one-minute spot on the Super Bowl can cost as much as one million dollars, not counting the cost of producing the commercial, which can run into the hundreds of thousands of dollars. (If there is a celebrity endorsement, the costs are even more.)

Advertising rates on local UHF stations are much less, but are still prohibitive for most small businesses. Even the smallest broadcast television stations have far too great a reach to be of much value to a beauty salon. There is too much waste and the cost is too high for the results you're likely to get. Broadcast television can not be considered a good buy for beauty salons.

Cable television differs from broadcast television in that the signals are transmitted by cable companies from powerful antenna systems to television receivers hooked up to that company's system. The service is offered through subscription, and viewers pay a basic monthly fee for a package that consists of a wide variety of channels. In addition to the normal channels, most cable companies offer premium channels at extra cost.

The value of cable television for advertisers is the medium's ability to target audiences much more specifically than broadcast television. Thus, cable TV, which some people refer to as "narrow-casting," offers a much wider choice of channels and programming devoted to very specific interests. For example, you can find a channel devoted solely to weather forecasts, one for medical information, one for news, one for sports, and so forth. In addition, most cable television companies offer community service channels, in which small communities can air their own programs, such as local high school football games. Some cable channels serve as video billboards, featuring nothing but a series of short print advertisements with musical accompaniment.

Because of the medium's ability to reach smaller, more highly targeted audiences and the lower costs for advertising, cable television is a better buy for a small business, such as a beauty salon, than broadcast television. This is especially true if the advertising runs on a community program channel or a video billboard channel. However, make the choice carefully. You probably will still be better served by print and radio than by television.

Direct Advertising

Media advertising, whether print or broadcast, utilizes a shotgun approach to reaching audiences. It is aimed to spread out and reach a demographic segment, without being very specific about individuals. It is the ideal way to target advertising when you know the general characteristics of your audience, but you can't identify them by name and address.

Direct advertising is ideal when you can identify specific groups or individuals. It provides a rifle, rather than a shotgun, approach to reaching audiences. You can tailor your message and approach to better appeal to different audience segments and set limits on the size and scope of the advertising effort. Therefore, direct advertising is usually less expensive than media advertising, yet it can be highly effective for a beauty salon.

DIRECT MAIL   Direct mail advertising involves nothing more than developing a letter or promotional piece describing your services and the benefits, and then mailing it to a preselected audience. This is an effective and inexpensive way to keep awareness high among your existing customers and to reach out with a personal message to new prospects. That's one reason you build a mailing list. You can gather other names and addresses from client recommendations and from other businesses. In some cases, you might be able to trade lists with other noncompeting businesses for names and addresses in the neighborhood you service. Once you've developed your list, keep it up-to-date.

The cost is relatively low. You pay for printing the piece and for postage. Because it is a targeted communication, your return should be reasonable. But the message has to aim at the needs of the audience. As with any advertising communication, stress the benefits, then tell the readers how the services you offer will help them.

Include the information they need to make a purchasing decision. You might want to add a coupon for a special sale or other inducement. Don't forget to include your name, address, hours of operation, and telephone number.

The direct mail piece you send must be attractive and command attention. It is competing with all of the other direct mail the audience receives, so you want to make sure it will intrigue them enough to open and read it. Here too, frequency is important. Make frequent mailings. Once a month is not too much. You can also do a direct mail campaign whenever you have something new to offer.

CIRCULARS Circulars, or printed sheets advertising your services, are another form of direct advertising. This involves developing and printing the circular, then hiring someone to distribute them in the neighborhood you've targeted. Like direct mail, this is a relatively inexpensive method of advertising. Its advantage is that you are reaching an area without knowing the people's names. Thus, it can extend your reach beyond that of your mailing list.

The message is important. Like any advertising, you have to first capture the readers' attention, then give them the benefits of your services. Limit the size of the circular to one side of a standard size paper. Use colored stock to attract attention, but make sure the piece is readable. Again, don't forget your name, address, hours of operation, and telephone number.

COOPERATIVE MAILINGS Cooperative mailings consist of stacks of small mail pieces from a number of companies, bundled together and mailed to occupants in various neighborhoods. These present a good opportunity to reach a large number of people in an area. The cost varies with the size of the mailing and the complexity of your particular advertisement. The advantage is that you are sharing costs with every other advertiser in the mailing. These mailings can be an effective advertising tool for your salon.

There are a number of firms that specialize in these mailings. To find the one servicing your area, ask your advertising agency, check your local telephone directory, or ask other business owners if they're using such a service. Also, pay attention to the direct mail advertising that comes into your home. The odds are that you are receiving one or more of these cooperative mailings yourself. Open them up and look through them. They usually contain information on contacting the mail service. While you're looking, note how the other ads are made. See what message they give and what style they take. Use the experience to get some ideas for your own advertising.

The firms that do the cooperative mailings will also print the pieces and provide the mailing list. In many cases, they will also help you develop your message. As with other media, keep your message oriented to the user. Stress the benefits and give the necessary information, including your salon name, address, hours of operation, and telephone number. You may also have a special offer as part of the mailing as an inducement to come into the salon for the first visit.

NEWSLETTERS   You might consider developing your own newsletter, your own salon newspaper that you mail periodically to your customers and others on your mailing list. The advent of relatively low-cost desktop publishing programs for personal computers makes this a very feasible task. Although it can take some time to put a newsletter together, the cost is fairly low and it is an effective means of keeping your salon name and services in front of your clientele. The costs involved are for printing and for mailing the newsletter. You may also have to pay someone for its preparation, if you don't have the writing or graphics skills to do it yourself.

Newsletters work well because they address items of interest to your clients and promote the image of your salon as progressive and modern. But, like any advertising medium, they must be done properly. The newsletter should have a masthead—an identification panel that contains the name of the newsletter, the date, and issue—and identification for your salon. Include items about your salon; for example, you can feature a particular service in each issue. In one newsletter, you could describe a facial, discuss the benefits, and talk about your esthetician. In the next issue, you could describe the benefits and features of your manicuring services. You might also want to profile one of your employees in each issue, describing his or her skills, background, and what benefits he or she brings to your salon. You probably should not discuss anything about your clients, however, as that could get very sensitive.

Use the newsletter to announce new services and new products you will offer and include notices of demonstrations or sales you will hold. Also include beauty industry items you think might be of interest to your clients, such as new products coming on the market and fashion trends. You can get this information from the trade magazines, but don't just copy the items. Take the information and write the article yourself. If you want to reproduce any item you see in a magazine, obtain the editor's permission and credit the source of that item in your copy. Ask your suppliers for information you can use in your newsletter.

You might also add black-and-white illustrations and photos to give it more eye appeal and better explain the subject matter. Your suppliers may be able to supply some of these, as well.

It may be possible to defray the costs of producing and mailing the newsletter by offering to include news items from other businesses in your area at a small fee. The businesses you approach, however, should be somewhat related to the beauty and fashion industry and should not be in competition with you. For example, the local bridal salon or flower shop would be good candidates, but the neighborhood saloon would not be suitable. This is an opportunity for these businesses to increase their customer base, so they ought to be interested in letting your clients know about new things happening in their businesses. They might also give you the names and addresses of some of their customers to supplement your mailing list. Just be careful not to overdo items from other businesses. You don't want to dilute the focus of your newsletter or let it get too far afield from your primary beauty business.

The newsletter doesn't have to be long. It can be anything from one page to many pages. Make it as long as it has to be to say what you want to say. Publish it as often as you have material to fill it. If you can publish your newsletter monthly, that's fine. But if you only publish it every other month or quarterly, that will work, too. And get feedback from your clients. Ask them how they like the newsletter, whether it's interesting and valuable to them. And ask them for suggestions about what they would like to see printed in it.

Publicity

Publicity is a valuable advertising and promotional tool that serves as an adjunct to your media advertising. The best part is that it is free. It is also very credible, because it is a third party endorsement of your salon. That is, someone else is saying good things about you. You're not saying them about yourself.

Newspapers, especially smaller local papers, are always looking for good, interesting, newsworthy items to print. Whenever you have something that may be newsworthy, for example, a new service being offered or an industry award that you've won, write a short publicity release and send it to the newspapers. If local magazines service your area, send the releases to them, too.

Keep the news releases short, simple, and factual. Answer the questions who, what, where, when, and why. Put the most important facts down first and expand on them in following paragraphs. Include a glossy black-and-white photo if you have one available. Stick to the facts, and don't engage in puffery or self-aggrandizement. On the top of the release, provide your name and telephone number so the editor can contact you for more information. Send the releases to the news editor whose name you can get from the newspaper.

There is no guarantee that the newspapers or magazines will print your news release. They are under no obligation to do so, and don't insult the editors by pointing out that you advertise in the newspaper. That won't make any difference. If the item is newsworthy and fits their needs, and if it is reasonably well written and professionally presented, they will use it. It is important that the release be presented in a professional manner. This means it should be grammatically and stylistically correct and should be neatly typed, double-spaced, on one side of standard size paper. If you haven't the ability to write good, clear English sentences, by all means, hire someone to write the releases for you. Either see your advertising agency or check with your local high school or college English departments for a freelance writer.

Other Advertising Media

In addition to the various advertising media previously discussed, there are other forms that you should be aware of. Some of these are quite valuable for a small service business; others are not so valuable, but you should have some idea of what they are.

OUTDOOR ADVERTISING   Outdoor advertising includes billboards and posters. Billboards are large advertising displays strategically located along roads and highways to capture the attention of drivers as they pass by. They are a valuable part of the advertising mix for large businesses that cover a wide area, but are not so useful for a small service business, such as a beauty salon. Billboards are expensive and can't target specific audiences as readily as other media. In addition, it is necessary to purchase space on many billboards to make sure enough of the right people see it. The only time a billboard should be considered for a beauty salon is if you are promoting a large multi-outlet chain operation. Some salon franchises utilize this type of advertising.

Posters are large printed cards that carry an advertising message. They are placed on flat surfaces, such as fences and walls, in the area they are meant to cover. While they may be fairly inexpensive to print, they may not be very effective for a service business. It is getting harder and harder to find legal places to put up posters. In addition, it is necessary to scatter them over a wide area to get sufficient coverage. Like billboards, they can't do a very good job of targeting specific audiences. Except in rare cases, posters are not a good investment for your advertising dollars.

COMMUNITY BULLETIN BOARDS   Community bulletin boards offer a good opportunity to reach a large audience at little or no cost. These are the bulletin boards you see in supermarkets and other locations, and are designed to convey information about local businesses and events. Check with your local supermarket about availablity, cost, and the requirements for posting a notice about your salon.

ADVERTISING SPECIALTIES   Advertising specialties are the little items you purchase to give away to your clients, including matchbooks, key chains, pens, and calendars, and they cover a wide price range. The value of the item for the purchaser is that each piece contains the name of the business and other relevant information, such as the telephone number and a brief benefit statement.

These little give-away items can be a valuable source of advertising for the salon, provided they are chosen with care. Make sure you pick items that will actually be used by the persons who receive them, as the reason for distributing them is to keep your name in front of the customer. If the item just sits in a drawer, it won't do the job. For example, desk or wall calendars are relatively inexpensive items that lend themselves for Christmas or Chanukah gifts. The recipient will keep and look at them almost constantly for a full year, which makes calendars a very effective advertising specialty.

Almost any item, however, can be effective for you, as long as it has some relevance to your salon and will be used reasonably frequently. The space available for your advertising message varies with the size of the item. On a pen you might have room only for the salon name and telephone number, but on a calendar, you might have enough space for a benefit statement.

Advertising specialties are sold by firms that specialize in these items. The better firms offer counseling to help you choose the items that will best serve your needs. Get recommendations from other businesses in the area, or look in the telephone directory under Advertising Specialties.

COOPERATIVE ADVERTISING   Don't overlook the possibilities of cooperative advertising assistance. Many manufacturers offer their customers an advertising allowance if the firm utilizes the manufacturer's logo in their advertising. Although the companies do this most often in conjunction with telephone directory advertising, they will sometimes offer monetary assistance for advertising in other media. This can help defray your advertising costs while giving you the added advantage of being associated with a large, well-known company. Ask your suppliers about cooperative advertising funds that may be available from the manufacturers whose products you use. Find out how you can qualify, and take advantage of these offers. It's virtually free money, but you have to ask. The manufacturers won't necessarily volunteer the information.

If you are a franchise operation, your franchisor will probably have a wide variety of advertising and promotional assistance programs available. Make sure you know what they are and take advantage of them.

SALES PROMOTION

In a sense, all advertising is promotion of your business. However, there are many things you can do in addition to your advertising programs to promote your business and increase sales. With some imagination and effort, you can keep your salon name in front of people in the community, bring them into the salon, and convert them into customers. And you can help keep your current customers loyal.

Sales and Promotions

You can offer special sales to promote your services. When you introduce a new service, you might give a special price to first-time buyers of that service, either as a stand-alone offer or piggybacked onto another service. For example, suppose you are introducing electrolysis services. You could make an introductory offer of a lower price for the first treatment, or have a "buy one, get one free" promotion, regardless of whether the patron buys another service.

You could also offer another service free or at a lower price when a client buys a standard service, for example, a free makeover with a facial. In some cases, you might offer products free or at reduced prices with a service, such as a free makeup kit with a makeover. This is especially effective when you can get the products at a lower cost as part of a manufacturer's promotion.

Don't overdo sales. If you've priced your services properly, they should be acceptable and fair to your clientele. If you run sales too often, they may start to wonder about the fairness of your price schedule, or they might not come back until your next sale. Don't reduce the price too drastically. Try to at least cover your cost. Remember, when you have a sale, you're trading current revenue for future revenue.

Also, have specific goals in mind for the sale and a clear idea of what you want to accomplish. Think it through before you make the offer. Limit the sale's time, and don't let it run too long. Advertise the sale, and use a coupon or some item that the client has to redeem to take advantage of it. This will help you keep track of how well both the advertising and the sale worked. After the promotion is over, analyze the results. Did it meet your goals? If not, find out why. Use what you've learned to guide you in making further promotions.

Open Houses and Demonstrations

An informed consumer is more apt to purchase your services. Hold an occasional open house in your skin care salon, so people can come in and see what you have to offer. Hold demonstrations to explain the benefits and features of your services, and show the people what you're selling. You might even have a guest speaker to talk about beauty and health, current fashion, or any relevant subject. Make it a party atmosphere. Have light, nonalcoholic refreshments, door prizes, and make sure each person gets a small gift—an advertising specialty item that has your salon name and telephone number on it. Have members of your staff on hand to answer questions.

Schedule the open house for a day or evening that you are not normally open. Open the affair to invited guests, only. If you know your audience, choose your guest list accordingly. Send invitations by mail, and request a response so you can get an idea of how many people will come. Let the size of your facility determine how many people you can accommodate, and don't overcrowd. You want the people to be able to mill around without being uncomfortable.

Get your suppliers involved, either to provide a speaker or to help with decorations. Many suppliers will be happy to give you some promotional help, so talk to them when you start making your plans. They should be able to give you some good ideas.

Tie-in Promotions

Make promotional deals with other businesses in your area, for example, your local bridal shop. Let them promote your services for you in exchange for a piece of the profits generated by their customers. For example, the bridal shop might send brides in for a facial and makeover the day before or the morning of the wedding. Similarly, you might promote the bridal shop to your clients who are getting married.

Visit dermatologists in the area. Explain your skin care services and show how you can help the doctor's clients with deep pore cleansing. Try for a relationship with the dermatologist, where he or she will refer patients to your salon and you will refer clients to his or her practice. Don't be afraid to try this. Dermatologists know the value of clean, healthy skin and many will be receptive to some kind of tie-in.

Limit your tie-in deals to businesses that are relevant to your salon. There should be some reason their clients might utilize your services. The tie-in has to be a good deal for both sides, so don't attempt to take any unfair advantages.

Community Service

Get involved in your community, and take part in community activities. Offer your services in charitable causes. For example, give a facial as a prize for the church bazaar, or donate a makeover as a prize for your local PBS station fund raising. Offer to be a speaker on skin care and health at your local high school or church.

In addition to keeping your name in front of the community, you'll also be giving something back to the community. But it is important to keep the focus of these activities on the help you're giving, not on what you'll get from it. Be careful not to give the perception that you're only doing these things for your own benefit.

SUMMARY

Marketing, advertising, and promotion are essential to the success of your business. Marketing is creating a demand for your services among your prospective clients. You have to let them know you are in business and that you have something of value to offer to them.

Start with a marketing communications plan that identifies your audience, the competitive situation you face, your strengths and weaknesses, and states your objectives and how you plan to meet them. The plan should contain the marketing information, your objectives, the message and positioning strategies, the tactics you will take to achieve them, measurement procedures, and your budget.

Advertising is one of your marketing tools. To be effective, it must attract the attention of the prospective clients, inform them of the services you offer and their benefits and features, and it must entice them to come into your salon.

Both the message and the media are important. You must choose the right media to reach your target audience, then communicate a message that leads the prospects to making a decision. The message must first catch their attention. It must be oriented to their needs and stress the benefits of your services. The message should position your salon in the minds of the prospective clients. Offer proof statements for the benefits, then close the sale by making the offer.

Advertising costs money. To make sure you are getting the best value for your advertising dollars, you must have some means of measuring the results. Know your effective cost per exposure figures. The most important measure of advertising effectiveness, however, is how many people responded to the advertisement and how much actual business it generated. Make sure you know how each new customer found your salon.

Unless you are an expert in advertising, you should work with an agency. Look for a small advertising agency that specializes in working with small businesses. Choose your agency with the same care you used in choosing your accountant and attorney.

There are many types of advertising media, each of which has advantages and disadvantages. Some are more useful for your salon business than others. You should utilize a number of advertising media to achieve your goals. One medium will not be sufficient.

Word-of-mouth advertising is one of the most effective means available. Satisfied customers who spread the word about your salon have outstanding credibility. And this medium is free, as long as you do a good job of satisfying your customers.

Print media, newspapers and magazines, may also be useful. Newspaper advertising is especially useful for the salon. You may use local daily newspapers, but don't overlook the local weekly papers or shopping journals. You can use either display ads or classified ads, depending on your purpose. Magazine advertising is normally not useful for a salon. They are expensive and their reach is too broad to be cost effective. However, your area may have some small, locally oriented magazines that you could consider. Telephone directory advertising is important but has a different purpose than other print media advertising.

Broadcast media can also be useful. Radio, in particular, can help attract new business at a relatively low cost. Network television is prohibitively expensive, although some cable TV networks offer competitive rates for small service businesses.

Direct advertising methods will also be useful in advertising your salon, especially when you can identify your prospects. Direct mail involves sending a letter or promotional piece to each of your prospects. Circulars which someone can distribute in your neighborhood are also useful. As with any advertising, however, the message you use is important and must meet the needs of your audience.

Other direct advertising methods include cooperative mailings and newsletters. Having your own newsletter that you mail out to your customer list and to prospects can keep your salon in the minds of the audience. Don't overlook publicity. Send news releases to the local media when you have some newsworthy item about your salon.

You could also utilize outdoor advertising like billboards, but these are usually too expensive to be cost effective. However, you might utilize community bulletin boards. Consider using advertising specialties, items such as key rings and calendars, that you give away to your clients.

Constantly promote your business. Use your imagination in keeping your salon in front of the community. You might run special sales, but have specific goals in mind for the sale and limit the time. Give open houses and demonstrations to show people what you can do. Make promotional deals with other businesses in your area. Finally, get involved in your community. Become a good citizen of the community.

SANITATION AND SAFETY
IN THE SALON

CHAPTER
SIXTEEN

For the salon owner, sanitation and safety are of paramount importance. Sanitation prevents disease, an important consideration when working on the skin, body, or nails. To understand sanitation, you should understand bacteria and how they can affect health, and you should be aware of the workings of the immune system in the body. You must know what factors cause and lead to the spread of disease and how to control or eliminate them.

In the course of daily operations, you and your employees come into contact with a variety of chemical substances, water, sharp implements, and machines that generate heat. Everyone in the salon should know how to handle these materials effectively and safely. Also, many of the services you perform generate waste materials, so you must know how to properly dispose of these.

Many of the sanitation and safety procedures are mandated by local, state, and federal government rules and regulations, which are discussed in Chapter 6. Review this chapter. You must be aware of and comply with these various laws. Failure to obey these rules can result in penalties, ranging from fines to loss of licenses, and ignorance of the laws is not an excuse.

PREVENTION OF INFECTIOUS DISEASES

The prevention of infectious diseases in your salon should be uppermost in your mind. Infectious, or contagious, diseases are spread from one person to another through contact. To prevent the spread of these diseases, avoid that contact and maintain scrupulous cleanliness and sanitary procedures and standards. The salon cosmetologist should never work on a client who has an obvious infectious disease, but refer that client to a physician. As a matter of good professional practice, he or she should promptly wash and sterilize all equipment used during a service and promptly place used materials in covered waste receptacles.

Cosmetologists must be aware of other diseases that may not be so evident, including AIDS, or Acquired Immune Deficiency Syndrome. The AIDS virus kills T-lymphocytes, rendering the immune system helpless and leaving the body prey to a wide variety of infections and diseases. The virus is transmitted through blood or other body fluids, usually either through sexual contact or sharing of needles. The chance of transmission of AIDS by any other means, according to the Center for Disease Control, is small.

Although the risk is small, during some services the employee can come into contact with the client's blood. At these times, the employee may want to consider using latex rubber gloves, even though his or her sense of touch may be slightly diminished. He or she may also consider wearing a surgical mask during some of the procedures.

SANITATION

The importance of sanitation in stopping the spread of disease was little understood, even by the medical profession, until the middle of the nineteenth century. In 1850, Ignaz Semmelweis, a German physician, was able to stop a series of fevers in his hospital by the simple expedient of having the doctors wash their hands before touching their next patients. In 1861, Louis Pasteur proved that germs cause disease and made a number of discoveries that helped prevent diseases. Since then, great advances have eliminated many serious diseases that were deadly scourges generations ago. Polio and diphtheria, for example, diseases that crippled or killed thousands of victims, have been virtually eradicated through the use of vaccines.

Even with these medical advances, however, sanitation is no less important today. The practice of proper sanitation procedures is vital to the success of your salon. The salon and all tools and implements used by the technicians must be kept spotlessly clean. The technicians must wear clean clothing and make sure that their hair and body are clean, also. Hands should be washed with soap and hot water and sanitized with alcohol before beginning work on a client.

Sanitation has two phases: sterilization, killing existing bacteria and viruses, and prevention, keeping new germs from growing. Towels and smocks must be washed in detergent and hot water and then stored in a closed, dry area. Implements must be washed in hot, soapy water, rinsed or wiped with alcohol after use, and stored in a dry sanitizer, a closed cabinet containing a fumigant or an ultraviolet light source.

Sterilization may be accomplished through the use of heat, ultra-violet light, gamma radiation, or chemicals. Heat may be moist, as in boiling or steaming, or dry, as in baking. High heat is effective in killing germs, but it may have an adverse effect on many implements, especially those made of plastic. Steam sterilization is usually carried out in an autoclave, an instrument that combines steam with high pressure. Short-wave ultraviolet light is effective in killing germs and is used in commercially available dry cabinet sanitizers and industrial germicidal lamps. Gamma radiation is also an effective germicide, but the equipment required is large and expensive, so its use is limited to the medical field.

Chemical sterilizing agents include fumigants, antiseptics, and disinfectants. Fumigants are chemical fumes that have the ability to kill germs. Antiseptics and disinfectants are liquid or dry chemical germicides that differ only in degree. Antiseptics are generally milder than disinfectants and can be used safely on the skin. Isopropyl alcohol (99 percent), boric acid, hydrogen peroxide (3 percent), sodium hypochlorite (bleach), and some soaps are commonly used antiseptics. Quaternary ammonium compounds (quats), formaldehyde, ethyl alcohol (70 percent), cresol, and phenol are commonly used disinfectants. Formaldehyde and formalin, a formaldehyde derivative, have been popular disinfectants for salon use. Formaldehyde has been suspected as a carcinogen, but recent studies indicate that it is safe, as long as it is used carefully. When using any chemical product, read and follow the manufacturer's instructions.

State cosmetology boards and local health departments should be consulted for recommendations on safe and effective germicides for use in the salon. Manufacturers' instructions for commercial germicides should be followed.

SANITARY AND WASTE DISPOSAL PROCEDURES

Proper sanitary and waste disposal procedures are also important. During the course of many services, the cosmetologist generates a considerable amount of waste, both recyclable and disposable. These waste materials must be handled safely and efficiently to avoid risk of contamination.

Reusable cloth items, such as towels and smocks, should be placed in a closed container after use. These items should be washed in hot water, dried with heat, folded, and stored in a closed cabinet or dry sterilizer until used again (Figure 16-1). Reusable metal or plastic

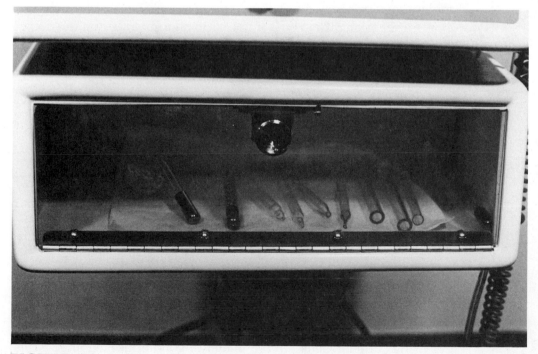

FIGURE 16-1   Dry sanitizer (Photo courtesy of Universal Techniques, Inc.)

implements should be washed in hot soapy water and sterilized with alcohol or other disinfectant after use, then stored in a dry or fumigant sterilizer.

Where feasible, disposable rather than reusable items should be used. For example, when giving a facial or applying makeup, it is more sanitary to use disposable bonnets, which are discarded after use on one client, than it is to wrap the client's head with towels (Figure 16-2). Disposable items should be placed in a closed trash receptacle immediately after use. Trash should not be allowed to accumulate in the salon, but should be periodically bagged in heavy duty plastic trash bags, tightly sealed, and disposed of according to local ordinances, either through municipal or private trash collection services or in legal landfills. The waste products generated in the salon will rarely be considered as hazardous. However, you should be especially cautious when disposing of used lancets or other sharp implements. These should be wrapped so they can't become a danger to anyone handling the trash.

When it comes to sanitation procedures, common sense should prevail. Most measures are obvious. Clean and sanitize chairs and implements after each client. Don't put products back in their containers after taking them out. If you drop an implement on the floor, pick it up immediately and wash and sanitize it before using it again. Wash and sanitize hands before and after each client. Sweep, scrub, and disinfect floors as needed. Wash the windows and mirrors frequently. Clean and dust the walls as needed. Keep the salon spotlessly clean. Establish a definite cleaning schedule, and follow it.

SAFETY IN THE SALON

Safety must also be a key concern in your salon, for both your clients and your employees. During the course of many services, the employee comes in contact with heat, water, steam, and electricity. He or she must be aware of the potential hazards involved with any of these. Heat and steam pose burn hazards; water can cause slipping; electricity can be a shock hazard. The cosmetologist must keep the client and himself or herself safe.

Safety is largely a matter of awareness—of being safety conscious and using common sense. It is a matter of good housekeeping. Spills should be wiped up as soon as they occur, before anyone can slip and

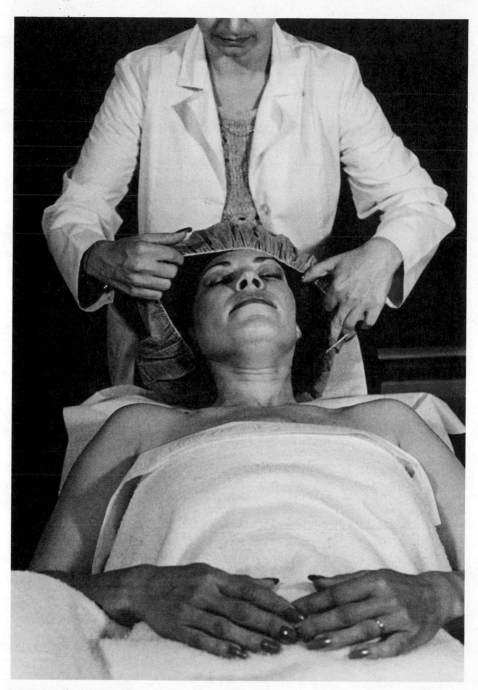

FIGURE 16-2 Use of the disposable bonnet

fall. Trash and debris should not be allowed to accumulate, but should be disposed of promptly and properly. Driers, heat lamps, vaporizers, and other heat sources should be monitored closely when in use so the client doesn't get burned. Lights should be covered to cut glare and as protection if the bulb should break. Passageways should be uncluttered to prevent accidents. All equipment should be maintained in good working condition. Burned out lightbulbs should be replaced quickly. All areas of the salon should be well lighted. Electrical circuits shouldn't be overloaded. Electrical machinery should be kept away from water to prevent short circuits. Keep a working flashlight handy to provide illumination in the event of a power failure.

Electrical circuits, whether in house wiring or in appliances, are protected against overloads by fuses or circuit breakers. When the current draw becomes too high for the circuit, the fuse blows before the wiring can overheat and cause a fire. Fuses are important safety devices. Don't use fuses that are too large for the circuit, and never bypass a fuse by inserting a metallic object into the fuse holder. Before replacing a fuse, determine the cause of the overload. When replacing a fuse, use a new fuse of the proper rating for the circuit.

Circuit breakers are resettable switches, designed to shut off when the permissible current draw is exceeded. Unlike fuses, which are destroyed in their function, circuit breakers are reusable.

Current can be either alternating or direct. Alternating current reverses polarity during a cycle. Direct current maintains the same polarity. Alternating current (AC) is usually developed by AC generators. Direct current (DC) is developed by batteries. Portable devices are often powered by direct current. Because alternating current can be transmitted efficiently over long distances, it is used for house current. Alternating current, however, cannot be stored; direct current can. Most electrical devices used in the salon rely on alternating current.

SUMMARY

In the salon, perhaps more than any other service business, cleanliness is paramount. You must be aware of laws that govern sanitation in salons and follow them to the letter. It is most important to prevent the spread of infectious diseases. Don't work on any client who has an infectious disease. Wash and sterilize all implements used during a service. Place all used materials into covered receptacles and dispose of waste properly.

Acquired Immune Deficiency Syndrome (AIDS) is a major factor today. The virus is transmitted through blood or other bodily fluids. While the risk of AIDS in the salon is small, you should still take precautions, especially when performing those services in which you may come into contact with the client's blood. Wear latex rubber gloves during these procedures.

Sanitation is important to stopping infectious diseases. Follow recommended sanitation procedures. Sterilize all instruments. Ask your state cosmetology board for recommendations, and use your common sense.

Safety is another concern. To keep your salon safe from accidents, use proper housekeeping. Be careful when handling or working around electricity, heat, steam, and sharp implements. Keep all machinery in good working order.

HELP FOR THE SMALL BUSINESS

CHAPTER

SEVENTEEN

It seems overwhelming. There's much to do, many details to look after, a lot of different things to consider. And the decisions are up to you. Make the right decisions and your business will prosper. Make the wrong ones and you court disaster. But, you're not an expert in all of the aspects of the salon business. How will you get the information you need? To whom can you turn for help? How will you make the right choices?

Don't despair. There is a lot of help available to you, if you know where to look for it. Virtually everyone you do business with, including the government, can provide some kind of assistance, so don't overlook any possibility.

This chapter discusses the types of assistance that are available to you as a small business owner or manager. Each section suggests sources where you can find that kind of help. Another valuable source for finding help is your own mailbox. As a registered business owner, you will receive mail from a variety of people who want to sell you something. Some will be offers for newsletter subscriptions, training courses, and seminars. Don't automatically discard such mail as "junk." Open and read every piece of mail that comes into your business. Granted, a lot of it will be useless, but you will find many offers that can help you run your skin care salon effectively and profitably. Investigate any that seem promising. Except for some precious time, it costs you nothing to investigate and evaluate any offer. What you find may, indeed, be well worth the effort you invested.

RESEARCH AND READING

You can get a lot of information on your own just from reading and doing your own research. Books and magazines covering almost every imaginable subject are readily available to you. Take advantage of them.

The Library

Your first stop should be your local library. Get to know the librarian, who can point you in the right direction to find critical information. Read as much as you can about business. There's a wealth of information in the library. There are hundreds of books on all aspects of business management. Browse through the section on business to see what's available. Then take stock of yourself. In what areas are you weak? You don't know anything about bookkeeping? Read an elementary book on the subject. You need to know about the law? Get a good business law book, but make sure it's not dated. Laws change, so be sure you're getting current information. You need to know the address and phone number of a trade association? Look it up in a directory of trade associations. The list could go on and on. You just have to do your homework.

Books and Magazines

Build your own reference library. In your office, you should keep a shelf of basic books to which you can refer when you need fast or recurring information. Include books on business law and management as well as professional reference books on the skin and body care services you offer.

Don't forget magazines. Consumer and trade magazines offer advice on business and professional matters. Look through the periodicals index in the library. Browse through your local bookstore, and examine some of the magazines that cover the information you need. Choose the best ones and subscribe to them. Don't limit yourself to magazines directed to general business subjects. The trade magazines that cater to the salon industry offer periodic business management tips.

When you see a book or magazine with information of value, buy it and read it. Make notes and underline relevant passages. Mark the passages so you can find them quickly. Make the reference work for you. Remember, all the information contained inside the book or magazine is useless to you if you never look at it.

Start a clipping file. When you read a newspaper or magazine article that has relevance to your business, cut it out and file it away for future reference. If you have any doubt about whether to keep an article, keep it. It's likely you'll need the information it contains at some point in the future.

Newsletters

Newsletters are an increasingly important method of business communication. A wide variety of newsletters is available covering a vast range of topics and coming from an equally broad variety of sponsors, from manufacturers to advocacy groups.

Some manufacturers of skin and body care products publish newsletters that describe new products and applications, industry news, and salon management tips and recommendations. The information they provide, though often slanted toward their products, can be very helpful. Some of these are free; others may be sold by subscription. Newsletters from advocacy groups, such as some health care providers, also provide a wide range of information relating to specific fields of interest. These publications can also contain many helpful tidbits of information that may be useful to your business.

Newsletters range in size from four pages to many times that amount and in frequency from weekly, monthly, and quarterly, to whenever the publisher manages to get an issue out. Most are sold on a subscription basis, with costs varying from a few dollars to many hundreds of dollars. In many cases, the information you'll glean from the publication will repay its cost many times over. Also remember that such publications, like the books and magazines you buy, are deductible as business expenses.

To get information on manufacturers' newsletters, call or write to the manufacturers of the products you use, or ask the distributors. For information on advocacy group or other newsletters, check with your librarian and look through a current directory of newsletters in the library's reference section. With any newsletter, ask for a sample copy before you subscribe.

Government Printing Office

One of your best sources of printed information is the Government Printing Office. This arm of the federal government offers a wide range of books, booklets, and pamphlets. Some are free. Some have a modest cost. For example, listed in the current catalog of publications is *The States and Small Business*. This is a directory designed to help business owners find sources of management information and assistance at the state level and costs $12.00. Also listed is *Financial Management: How to Make a Go of Your Business*. This seventy-nine-page paperback contains information required to familiarize the small business owner with the basic concepts of financial management and costs $2.50. You can also get census data from the GPO.

If you have a Government Printing Office bookstore in your city, pay it a visit and see what it has to offer. The GPO has a free catalog of books. Write to: Free Catalog, Government Printing Office, P.O. Box 37000, Washington, DC 20013-7000.

CONTINUING EDUCATION

You can also get help by going back to school. Throughout the country are many in-class educational opportunities for small business owners. You can attend adult evening education classes, college courses, and seminars or even take correspondence and videotape courses on a range of business subjects.

Adult Evening Classes

Quite a few community colleges and high schools around the country offer adult evening classes covering a variety of subjects, such as elementary bookkeeping, advertising for the small business, or computer basics. Many of these courses are designed for small business owners and managers and provide elementary to advanced information about business management topics. Classes are usually held one or two evenings a week for periods of up to ten weeks. The teachers are often experts in the field, who can answer your specific questions and offer advice in addition to the classroom instruction.

The cost of adult evening classes is usually minimal, requiring a relatively low fee, the cost of books and other materials, the time and interest on your part, and your willingness to do the work. For information on specific courses offered in your area, call your local board of education.

College Courses

In addition to adult evening classes, you might want to consider taking full semester college courses in specific subjects. These can include business administration subjects such as basic accounting, business law, or financial management. Or you might take courses in subjects that will help you with the services you'll offer in the salon, such as diet and health, nutrition, or public health services.

Colleges and universities offer full evening curricula leading to a degree. However, it is not necessary to enroll in a degree program. You can take individual courses without earning college credit. You won't get a grade, but you will gain the knowledge as long as you do the work.

College courses are comprehensive and cover a lot of information that will be of use to you. They are much more expensive than adult evening classes, however, since you will pay on a credit hour basis, the same as a matriculated student. In addition, they may be somewhat restrictive in that the qualifications for getting into a class will be more strict. You will probably have to meet certain educational standards and may have to take courses that are prerequisites to the class you want to attend. For information on course availability, costs, and entrance requirements, contact the admissions office of your local college or university.

Seminars and Training Courses

Attendance at seminars and training courses is an ideal method of acquiring information and knowledge. Although the terms are often used interchangeably, they are two different things. A seminar denotes a more or less informal discussion group in which all the participants contribute to and share in the dissemination of information. The participants are usually led by a seminar leader who directs the discussion. Panel discussions are a form of seminar. A training course, by contrast, is a classroom-like experience in which a lecturer teaches the participants. Before you sign up for a seminar or training course, make sure you know what the format is and what you'll be expected to bring to the meeting.

Seminars and training courses are generally shorter and more focused than college or adult evening classes. Seminars typically last from one hour to half a day, although some are longer, and are usually limited to a specific topic. Many seminars are held in conjunction with industry trade shows or association meetings and are scheduled to allow the participants to attend a number of sessions. Costs are variable, depending on the organization sponsoring the events, but are generally minimal.

Training courses are usually longer than seminars. They typically range from one day to as much as a week, although some are longer and some are shorter. Because of their short duration, their content is usually compressed and focused on a specific topic. Since they have to cover a lot of information in a short amount of time, they tend to be very intense and require a lot of concentration and attention. They tend to be more expensive than seminars and adult evening classes, though less expensive than college courses.

These gatherings are available in a wide variety of subject matter and sponsorship. Many cosmetology industry manufacturers offer training courses on the use of their products and on the latest techniques for specific services. Such training courses are ideal ways to keep abreast of current trends in your industry. Manufacturers are also expanding their offerings to include salon management topics.

As mentioned earlier, most trade associations and many organizations also offer training courses and seminars as an integral part of their meetings. The courses are usually spelled out clearly in their meeting prospectuses, so read these carefully when you receive them.

In addition, a number of institutions of higher learning offer seminars and training courses outside of their regular curricula, many of which are designed for small business owners and managers. Also, many private business and industry consultants offer training courses.

Independent Study

One of the values of participation in a classroom course or seminar is the chance to meet and talk with people in the same circumstances as you. You can sometimes learn as much from the informal give-and-take you get by talking with other small business owners and managers as you can from the course itself. But if you haven't the time or the inclination to attend classes, you can still go back to school through independent study by correspondence courses or videotaped

instruction. While you will lose the synergy developed through interaction with other students, you will still be able to acquire the basic
knowledge and information you need.

Correspondence courses hold an old and honored place in
American education. In essence, you learn by mail. The school supplies you with course materials, usually in the form of books and lesson plans, tests your knowledge at the end of each lesson, and gives a
final examination when you've finished all of the lessons. You study
at your own pace under the tutelage of one or more instructors with
whom you communicate by mail or telephone.

There are many correspondence schools, and they offer a wide
range of courses. Some are reliable; others are not. Before you sign up
for a course, investigate the school thoroughly. Read and understand
the course descriptions and the contract. These schools can sometimes
be expensive, so make sure the course meets your needs before you
sign up.

Videotape Instruction

Instructional materials on videotape are also available. These taped
mini-courses, developed by a number of universities and other organizations, cover a wide range of business-related subjects, from finance
and accounting to leadership skills, and vary in price. The tapes can
be an effective way of gathering information and knowledge. The format lets you watch at your convenience, and you can view the tape as
many times as you want. The disadvantage is the impersonality.
There is no interaction between you and the teacher. Instructional
videotapes are usually advertised in various trade and consumer
magazines.

ASSOCIATIONS AND ORGANIZATIONS

Like minds working together can accomplish many things that can't
be accomplished by one person working alone. Since the beginning of
time, people have been banding together to provide themselves with
mutual protection and collective advantage. Businesses are no different. Virtually every industry, whether manufacturing or service, is
represented by a trade association. Many retail and commercial areas
are represented by a merchant's association, and countless fraternal

and business organizations cross industry and business lines to help give a voice to the concerns of individual members of various groups. Such associations and organizations can be a tremendous aid to you and your salon, providing you with information and advice.

Trade Associations

Trade associations are organizations established to serve the collective needs of member businesses in a given industry. They are typically financed by dues and fees paid by the members and run by a salaried professional staff, governed by an executive board made up of elected representatives from the businesses. They are usually national in scope, with a number of state and local branches. There can be more than one trade association for any industry. The current edition of the *Encyclopedia of Associations,* for example, lists nine trade associations under the heading of Cosmetology.

These organizations offer an impressive array of services to their members. They keep members up-to-date on industry trends, conduct educational and public relations programs, and promote industry standards. In addition, they monitor legislative activity and lobby on behalf of the industry. Many also provide for group health and liability insurance coverage for member businesses, and some offer assistance in finding financing.

Some associations publish newsletters and magazines that are slanted toward the industry and contain many articles about salon management. Many associations also conduct an annual convention, complete with trade show exhibits and seminars and training courses. These are excellent opportunities for a salon owner or manager to keep up with industry trends and to increase knowledge about the field.

If you are in business, you'll find it worthwhile to join a trade association that provides invaluable services and advice. Get information from all the associations that service the beauty industry, and study the literature. Then join the one that offers the most benefit to you. Become active in the organization. Attend local monthly meetings and the national convention. Remember, dues and expenses you incur attending the meetings are deductible as business expenses.

Merchant Associations

Merchant associations, in contrast with trade associations, are small, local groups usually consisting of small retail and service business

owners in a given area. They are formed by the merchants in a neighborhood or shopping area and limit their activities to that area. They
are not allied with any given industry. Like trade associations, merchant associations look after the interests of their members. They are
not usually managed by a paid staff, but are run by committees
elected from the membership.

Merchant associations offer a number of activities. They can
provide support in tenant-landlord negotiations, lobby at the local
government level, and keep members informed about pending legisla-
tion that may affect small business operations in the area. They may
also organize neighborhood clean-up campaigns and other programs
to make sure the merchants are "good neighbors" in the locality.

Join your local merchant association, and take an active part in its
activities. The rewards can be substantial.

Fraternal and Service Organizations

Any number of other organizations can provide help to your salon.
These are organizations made up of people who share common interests and are not related to any industry. Some can give direct aid, for
example, the National Association for Female Executives that can provide financing to women who meet the credit requirements.

Most, such as service organizations like the Kiwanis or Rotary,
provide indirect help. They are ideal avenues for networking, that is,
establishing those informal relationships that you can call on for help.
Don't discount the value of networking. The people you meet and the
contacts you make can pay great dividends. By investing your time
and effort in a fraternal or service organization, you will develop a
fertile source you can mine for information and assistance. You'll also
be helping better your community. It is a good way for you to give
something back to the community in which you work.

THE GOVERNMENT

There are many people who feel that "government help" is a contra-
diction in terms. And it is true that dealing with a government
agency, on any level, can be a frustrating experience. The government
is more than just a body that promulgates laws, regulations, and
requirements, however. Through its various agencies, it is also a great
compiler of information. More important to the business owner,

though, is that these government agencies, especially at the federal level, will share much of that information willingly and freely—if you know where and who to ask for it.

At the federal level, you can get information and advice from a number of agencies. The Government Printing Office discussed earlier is just one example. Other agencies that can give you help include:

The **Small Business Administration** (SBA) offers a number of programs to assist small businesses and publishes a vast array of pamphlets and books on business subjects. These are available at little or no cost. The SBA also operates loan guarantee programs to help small businesses get financing. Contact your local SBA office and find out what programs they offer that can help you.

The **Department of Labor** can provide you with statistical information about the cosmetology industry and keep you abreast of the laws governing employment.

The **Food and Drug Administration** (FDA) is your best source to answer questions about the safety and efficacy of beauty care products and equipment. The agency publishes a monthly magazine, *The FDA Consumer,* that contains articles about health and safety issues. The magazine provides valuable information and is a worthwhile addition to your library. It would also make interesting reading for your clients.

The **Federal Trade Commission** (FTC) can give you information about business and industry practices. This agency is a good source for information about the rules and regulations that govern franchise operations.

The **Internal Revenue Service** (IRS) can keep you up-to-date on the tax laws that govern your salon. The agency publishes a number of free informational pamphlets that explain the tax laws and regulations.

Most states have similar agencies that can provide the same type of information and help, although on a more limited basis. At the state level, your most important agency will be your state board of cosmetology, which can apprise you of the laws and regulations governing salons in the state, answer your questions, and provide guidelines for your operation.

Regardless of the level of the government agency, however, keep in mind that it exists to help you. Don't be hesitant to ask for help and information when you need it. Your taxes pay for these services; it's up to you to utilize them. All of these government agencies are listed in major city telephone books. Look them up and make a file of those you are likely to call.

SCORE

You can get free advice and counsel on business matters from SCORE, the Service Corps of Retired Executives. This is a volunteer counseling group made up of experienced business executives who are either retired or still active in business. They donate their time to provide advice and guidance to small business owners. The group is sponsored by the SBA and its services are free.

There are SCORE branches in all major cities. They are listed in the telephone book, or you can call your local SBA field office for the location of the branch nearest to you. This is an excellent source of help. It can give you one-on-one guidance that you would be hard pressed to find anywhere else. If you do nothing else, you should take advantage of this service.

SUMMARY

Help is available to you, if you know where to look for it. It starts with your own research and reading. Visit your local library, which contains a wealth of information and advice, and learn how to use it. Start your own reference library. Have a shelf of basic books on business and on the services you offer. Read the trade magazines and clip articles you find useful. Subscribe to one or more industry newsletters. Get a catalog from the Government Printing Office and order books and pamphlets that offer information about business.

You might also consider going back to school. Many institutions offer classes and seminars on a wide range of business subjects. Seminars and training courses are available from a number of independent sources. If you don't have the opportunity to attend classes, look into buying videotapes or taking advantage of self-study courses.

Become active in your trade associations. They offer a wide range of help. Your local merchant's association can also be a source of information. Membership in fraternal and service organizations can introduce you to people who can help you.

The government also offers help to small business owners. Many agencies offer assistance. SCORE, a volunteer counseling group sponsored by the SBA, is an extremely valuable source of advice and information. These services exist for your benefit. Don't hesitate to use them.

INDEX

theft and misconduct insurance, 113
tools/equipment used by, 190–91
training, 177–78
see also Staffing
Employee's Withholding Allowance Certificate, 162
Employer Identification Form (EIN), 162
Employers, tax information for, 161–64
Employer's Information Return of Tip Income, 162
Employer's Tax Guide, 161
Employment Eligibility Verification Form, 162
Employment Taxes, 161
EPA (Environmental Protection Agency), 88, 92
Equal Credit Opportunity Act, 135
Equal Employment Opportunity Commission (EEOC), 88, 94–95
handicapped clients and, 214
Equipment, 39
body massage, 52–54
consultation room, 74
defined, 184
electrolysis, 57
employee, 190–91
facials, 52
hair removal, waxing and, 57
hydrotherapy treatments, 55
leasing, 189–90
makeup/cosmetic application, 59
management of, described, 183–84
manicuring, 60–61
purchasing, 184–89
retail services, 62
treatment room, 77
wraps/packs, 54
Equity
balance sheet and, 144
capital, sources of, 133–35
Esthetician, 159
Esthetics
business, 5–6
see also Business
defined, 5

Expenses
business, business plan and, 26
legal services, 104
management of, 148–51
taxes, 150–51
employer information, 161–64

F
Facials, 51–52
equipment for, 52
Facility
business plan and, 24–25
inspecting, 39
Fair Labor Standards Act, 93
FDA Consumer, 89–90
FDA (Food and Drug Administration), 88–90
continuing education and, 307
Federal agencies, 87–95
Federal Tax Deposit Coupon, 162
Federal Trade Commission (FTC), 88, 90
Disclosure Rule, 43
Federal Unemployment (FUTA) tax, 163
Fictitious name, 105
Finances
accounting, choosing, 119–20
bank, choosing, 120–22
business plan and, 23–28
obtaining, 27
sources of, 124–35
business, 127–35
personal, 125–27
Financial management
bankruptcy and, 152–54
bookkeeping/accounting and, 139–45
budgets/cash management and, 145–47
daily journal, 140–41
reconciliation, 228–29
discussed, 137–38
expense management and, 148–51
price management and, 147–48
taxes and, 150–51